AGELESS ATHLETES

THE SCIENTIFIC APPROACH TO ACHIEVING HIGH-LEVEL FITNESS AND COUNTERACTING THE EFFECTS OF AGING

RICHARD A. WINETT, Ph.D.

CB
CONTEMPORARY
BOOKS
CHICAGO · NEW YORK

Library of Congress Cataloging-in-Publication Data

Winett, Richard A. (Richard Allen), 1945–
  Ageless athletes.

  Bibliography: p.
  Includes index.
  1. Physical fitness.   2. Physical education and
training—Psychological aspects.   3. Athletes.
I. Title.
GV481.W58   1988   613.7′1   88-16186
ISBN 0-8092-4824-7

Published by Contemporary Books, Inc.
180 North Michigan Avenue, Chicago, Illinois 60601
Manufactured in the United States of America
International Standard Book Number: 0-8092-4824-7

Published simultaneously in Canada by Beaverbooks, Ltd.
195 Allstate Parkway, Valleywood Business Park
Markham, Ontario L3R 4T8 Canada

Photographs of the Zanes are by Jack Mitchell.

All other photographs were supplied courtesy of the athletes.

To the two lights of my life—
my wife, Sheila, and my daughter, Emily

Contents

Please Note

This book contains principles for optimizing motivation and performance, exemplar training routines, and current training routines of top masters athletes. Many of these routines include intense training sessions. These routines should not be attempted by novices, and even long-term athletes should not quickly and markedly escalate their training. Anyone considering a substantial change in their fitness and training activities should undergo a comprehensive physical examination.

Acknowledgments

The book could not have been written without the time and effort put into questionnaires, telephone interviews, and portrait drafts from all the athletes featured in this book. Let me say again, "Thank you!" I especially want to acknowledge Clarence Bass's encouragement over the years. He has given me that extra boost which has enabled me to extend myself in several successful endeavors. My friend Joe Germana has also been a great source of encouragement and support through all the ups and downs of the last few years. I also want to thank Cindy Koziol and Joy Weiss, who stuck by me through all the various drafts—all of which, of course, were needed "as soon as possible."

1
Foundation for *Ageless Athletes*

THE GENESIS OF *AGELESS ATHLETES*

About 30 years ago, when I was a small, weak, flabby, and shy 13-year-old, I decided to do something about my appearance and physical condition. I persuaded my parents to buy me a 110-pound barbell set.

I recall following the instructions that came with the set and struggling to complete 10 repetitions with 30 pounds in the standing press. A few weeks later, I was able to do 10 reps with 40 pounds. My progress and results continued to be orderly and visible, though never spectacular. However, here was something I could do reasonably well, alone if I wanted to, and where it was quickly evident that, as the adage says, "You got out of it what you put into it." In a word, I was hooked.

I continued training through high school, college, and graduate school in various gyms, and then eventually in my own small home gym. In the 1960s and even early 1970s, anyone continuing to train past adolescence was still an oddity and considered suspect. Of course, that started to change with the "running boom" and the increasing emphasis on health and wellness. In the late 1960s, I had become part of the trend by adding running to my own training regime.

By the late 1970s and early 1980s, the very things I had been doing for so many years were suddenly very in. It seemed that everyone was interested in how to combine weights, running, and other aerobics. In fact, a national magazine, *The Runner*, did a long feature on my "Total Training" approach.

Fitness and health promotion has shown some predictable hyperbole, fallout, and evolution during the last several years. For example, I really doubt that 50 percent to 60 percent of adults regularly exercise to any appreciable extent, as some surveys have suggested. I think the true figure may be closer to 20 percent. On the other hand, the variety of aerobic activities people are doing has expanded. Weight training seems a stable part of most fitness programs, and people are beginning to understand that health is a product of many interrelated factors such as diet, exercise, stress control, and interpersonal relationships.

Along the way, the sociocultural emphasis on fitness and health has created one phenomenon that is hard for anyone to ignore: the "older" athlete. The 35-year-old, 40-year-old, 55-year-old, 65-year-old, and even 75-year-old athlete is no longer considered a dilettante, or worse, a freak. Indeed, the older athlete is becoming the rule rather than the exception.

The middle-aged athlete may be like Carlos Lopez, 40, or Priscilla Welch, 43, who seem to be improving and pulling away from the pack at open, international 10K or marathon races. Or, older athletes may be like Kay Baxter or Albert Beckles, who at 46 and 57 respectively still compete at the highest level in bodybuilding. More likely, however, the older athlete is someone with more ordinary abilities who simply never stopped training (despite warnings of doom from friends and peers), or who picked up training again, or who just started in his or her middle years. No matter what level of ability and aspiration, we older athletes are daily redefining terms such as *middle-aged* and changing medical and social expectations about aging and performance.

To pick up my personal story again, in 1985, at the age of 40, I started to become intrigued with aging, performance, and masters athletes. (Masters athletes are generally considered to be over 40, although in some sports, masters are only over 35.) At the same time, it seemed fascinating not only to see how long I could continue to train at a "good level," but, more importantly, to find out if I could actually improve in strength and appearance from where I was in my 20s and early 30s.

Background Research on Aging and Performance

I gathered information on the subject of aging, athletics, and performance. The material I found could roughly be classified into five categories. In the first category were various theoretical and (usually) animal analog research studies about the aging process. Several biological positions on aging have been developed from this work, with both overlapping and sometimes contradictory points. To me, these papers were not very interesting. We all know that although people seem to age differently, we all do eventually get older. These papers, to be discussed a bit more at the end of this book, were not telling me much about performance in the face of the aging process nor how to optimize performance.

In a second category were studies best exemplified by Ralph Paffenbarger's well-known research on physical activity and longevity. The fact that physically active people live longer is not surprising, although it was nice to see that point documented. However, I was more interested in high-level performance, not so much the question of longevity per se.

In a third category, there were a few cross-sectional studies on aging, activity level, and performance. In cross-sectional research, you look at groups of people, differing on certain characteristics, at one point in time. For example, you can study active and inactive men's treadmill performances with groups of 40-, 50-, and 60-year-old men. Not surprisingly, these studies showed differences at different ages between active and inactive people. But they also showed a substantial drop-off in performance with age despite activity levels. These data are far from being optimistic, but they are not as conclusive as longitudinal data, especially well-executed longitudinal studies that follow the same people over time.

Another category of materials includes articles that started to appear in magazines, particularly running magazines, about masters athletes. Except for Mike Tymn's column in *Runner's World*, however, these articles were sporadic, and they were not interrelated. But they were certainly inspiring. Here you could get a good idea how some of the top masters runners were training, competing, and generally living their lives.

A final category contained only three entrants, but they were all helpful and exciting. Jan and Terry Todd, in their *Lift Your Way to Youthful Fitness* (Boston: Little, Brown, and Company, 1985), had a thoughtful section on aging and athletics and showed what a training program could do for previously sedentary middle-aged men and women. Lloyd Kahn's book, *Over the Hill—But Not Out to Lunch* (Bolinas, CA: Shelter Publications, 1986), portrayed about 50 well-known and some not so well-known over-40 athletes. Some of these were life-long athletes while others were individuals who only took up training in their middle years. The portraits were all interesting and nicely written with a personal slant on each person. However, I wanted to know much more about their training and what kept them going over many years.

By far the best material I ever read about masters athletes is a classic book by John Jerome called *Staying With It: On Becoming an Athlete* (New York: Viking Penguin, 1984). Mr. Jerome chronicled his own successful return to top-flight swimming in his middle 40s after a long hiatus of relative inactivity. Along the way, he covered in unique style many points about training, motivation, and the aging process.

The book remains one that should appear on any master athlete's bookshelf. What is particularly inspiring about the book is Mr. Jerome's development of a sophisticated approach to training that allowed him not only to compensate for some effects of aging (e.g., stiffness, slower recovery), but also to surpass competitive swim times he had made in high school and college.

From these books and other materials, I started to distill my own ideas for the emphasis and content of a book about masters athletes, *Ageless Athletes*.

Training, Aging, and Fitness

One of my first tasks in formulating my approach to this book was to develop a better idea—beyond assuredly exciting anecdotal accounts such as John Jerome's—about what may be expected if a person seriously trained in middle age. This does not mean people who "exercised or kept fit," but individuals who continued to be dedicated athletes.

As I noted before, the cross-sectional studies all pointed to a rather marked "inevitable decline" with aging. Some of the active people I knew or saw around me at the large university where I worked seemed to defy this idea about inevitable decline.

The Impact of Training

One small longitudinal study on athlete performance and aging was available to help explain the difference between the studies and what I observed. The unique and provocative longitudinal data were collected by Dr. Michael L. Pollock and his associates. There are a few other longitudinal studies in the literature, but even with its limitations, this is the best one. Most of the prior research on aging and fitness was cross-sectional and had not taken into account either life-style or training factors. When these factors *were* considered in the samples studied, it became obvious that training levels almost invariably declined with age. Thus, from this research it has not been possible to understand *what amount of reduced fitness was attributable to age and what amount was attributable to reduced training.*

Dr. Pollock has extensively studied 24 healthy, active men, ages 50–82, who continued to train. The men were first tested between 1971 and 1974 and then again about 10 years later. All of the men at one point were highly respectable master aerobic athletes, mostly runners. At both points of testing, the men received state-of-the-art physical, cardiovascular, and body composition examinations. What makes Pollock's data so important is that through questionnaires and interviews it was also possible to document quantity and quality of aerobic training and the addition of strength, flexibility, or alternate aerobics to the training regime on a year-to-year basis.

The men in Pollock's study were classified into two groups: competitive and postcompetitive. The competitive group continued to train for high-level competition. They maintained a training pace within 30 seconds per mile of their pace 10 years earlier. The postcompetitive group was no longer training for competition. Their pace was now 90 seconds slower per mile than when first tested. Thus, the competitive group closely maintained training intensity, while the postcompetitive group markedly reduced training intensity.

Interestingly, both groups maintained the volume of their training. At the first testing, the competitive runners trained about 36 miles per week compared to about 34 miles per week at the second testing. For the postcompetitive group, the figures were about 27 miles per week compared to about 23 miles per week.

TABLE 1

Physical Characteristics and Cardiovascular, Body Composition, and Health-Related Measures of Competitive and Postcompetitive Athletes at Test 1 and Test 2, 10 Years Later

| | Competitive | | Postcompetitive | |
	Test 1	Test 2	Test 1	Test 2
Age	50.2	60.0	53.9	62.4
Height	5'8.5"	5'8.5"	5'10.25"	5'9.5"
Weight	148.5	146.7	158.8	155.5
$VO_{2 max}$ (ml · kg^{-1} · min^{-1})	54.2	53.3	52.5	45.9
Max Heart Rate	177	170	170	163
Percent Fat	11.6	13.6	14.3	16.3
Thigh Girth	21.3"	21.7"	21.5"	21.3"
Bicep Girth	12.3"	12.0"	12.0"	11.9"
Waist Girth	31.8"	32.3"	32.4"	33.6"
Rest Heart Rate	47.6	42.0	50.5	51.9
Systolic Blood Pressure (mmHg)	117	118	127	138
Diastolic Blood Pressure (mmHg)	80	79	79	80

Table 1 shows some key characteristics of the two groups at the two testing times selected from Dr. Pollock's data presented in his 1987 *Journal of Applied Physiology* article. The most intriguing data on this table show that:

- The competitive group remained at a lower body weight.
- The competitive group maintained VO_2 max while the postcompetitive group declined. (VO_2 max is the abbreviation for the maximum rate at which an individual can consume oxygen during a physical activity. According to Brooks and Fahey, 1984, p. 9, "One definition of physical fitness is VO_2 max.")
- Maximum heart rate declined for both groups, but still remained higher for the competitive group.
- Both groups increased in percent body fat, but the competitive group remained lower.
- Both groups showed a decrease in bicep size and an increase in waist size (particularly the postcompetitive group), while thigh size slightly increased in the competitive group and slightly decreased in the postcompetitive group.
- The competitive group showed a reduction in resting heart rate while the postcompetitive group stayed about the same.
- Diastolic blood pressure remained about the same for both groups, but systolic blood pressure increased for the postcompetitive group and remained about the same for the competitive group.

Implications of the Study

These data certainly indicate that when training intensity is maintained, many indicators of fitness can be maintained. This major finding is more graphically shown in Figure 1 (page 8). This figure, based on a figure in the same journal article, presents composite data from many studies that compare the VO_2 max of athletic, lean men with overweight, untrained men across years. On the graph there are also the data from Dr. Pollock's study. Here you can clearly see that athletes maintain a much superior VO$_2$ max to untrained individuals across the ages 35 to 75. Although there is a decline with age, the 70-year-old athlete is still superior to the untrained 35-year-old, a fact that has great individual and public health significance.

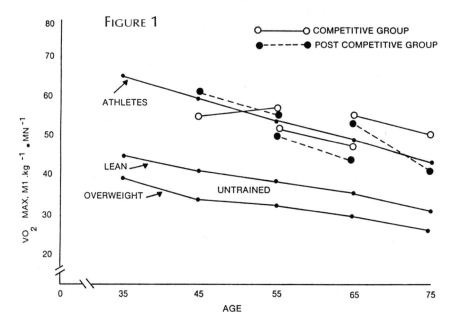

The postcompetitive group closely followed the decline for VO$_2$ max of the typical athlete. But, also note that the competitive group aged about 55 at the second testing remained stable. Those aged 65 at the second testing showed only a slight decline, and the most elderly competitive group showed some decline at about 75 years but remained well above the typical elderly athlete.

The body composition data is also very intriguing (Table 1). Both groups appeared to be increasing in percent body fat and losing upper body size (bicep girth size). However, these findings may not be directly caused by aging, but rather *how* these individuals trained. For example, there was no loss in muscle mass in their legs (thigh girth size). This finding is expected given the specificity of training. Only three of the men did any regular upper body training. Two were involved in weight training and one was a cross-country skier for about a third of each year. These men were the only ones to maintain their percent body fat. Age was apparently not a factor since one man was in the 50–59 age category, one 60–68, and one 69–78. Thus, the type of training may influence outward appearances of aging. For example, continuance of weight training may maintain lean body mass and upper body size.

As a research scientist, I know that a good deal of caution is needed when interpreting the data from Dr. Pollock's study. For example, when you look at Table 1, it is apparent that there were some differences between the competitive and post-competitive athletes at the first testing. This is known as *selection bias*, an almost inevitable aspect of this kind of research. However, at this point, Dr. Pollock's work is apparently all we have in the way of longitudinal data. And, overall, it appears clear that keeping training intensity high is a real key to maintaining high-level fitness and possibly other indicators of health.

At a minimum, it can be concluded that for those people willing and able to keep training hard, there will not be great performance drop-offs. For some sports, athletes in their 40s and 50s may show little or no signs of deteriorating performance, and maybe, just maybe, some athletes can actually improve in their middle years.

A Personal Test

Armed with this information, I decided to do something about my own training to see how far I could progress. Over the years, while I have always continued weight training, I have gone through six distinct "incarnations." When I was a teenager, becoming large and bulky was considered the ideal. Taking that to heart, I lifted and ate my way up to almost 190 pounds. With a medium frame at about 5'7", I was enormous. I was quite strong, but my bulk was mostly fat.

Through the urging of some friends, I slimmed down to about 165 pounds and focused more on bodybuilding. I trained about four to five times per week for a weekly total of about seven hours. When I was 21, the picture of me that you see here took second place in a national contest sponsored by the old *Strength and Health* magazine.

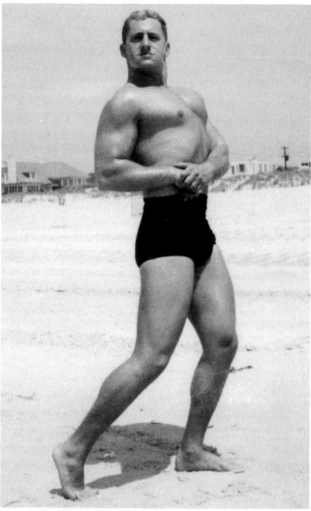

The author at twenty-one in a picture that took second place in a *Strength & Health* magazine contest.

For about the next ten years, I usually did only two short high-intensity weight workouts a week, plus jogging two to three miles, three times a week. During this time, I never looked in very good condition for a simple reason—I wasn't.

Not surprisingly, my next venture took me into running. Although I still continued my two weight workouts per week, I also ran up to six days per week. I did everything—overdistance, fartlek, intervals, and hard-easy days. In looking back over my running and weight training records from that eight-year period, the evidence in black and white is hard to refute. Of course, I got weaker in my weight training, but over time and after all those miles, I also got slower! I now believe that if I had just run shorter distances, or if I had only concentrated on running fast intervals for a few miles three times per week, I would have done much better. Running a fraction of the mileage but more intensely, I think, would have made me fitter and faster. It also would have been a lot more enjoyable.

About the time I was becoming less interested in running, I started to correspond with Clarence Bass. Clarence is a lawyer in Albuquerque, a former national level Olympic lifter, and a champion masters bodybuilder. He has also written the best training and nutrition books I have ever read (see pages 102 to 113 for a profile of Clarence).

Through Clarence's instruction, encouragement, and example, I started to diversify my training. I first substituted some other aerobic activities (an Air Dyne and rowing machine) for my "easy" running days and adopted a hard-easy system for my weight training days. I next reduced my running to no more than two days per week and five miles at a time, did my other aerobics on two other days, and worked out on an every-other-day split routine for weight training. During this time, I also greatly upgraded and expanded my home gym. I lost about five pounds, reduced the fat in my diet, and started to train following a first generation of the periodization system to be described in Chapter 3.

The next picture of me shows that this overall approach worked reasonably well. At 41, I had equalled or exceeded most of the weights I had used 10 to 20 years earlier, but now I was at a much lower body weight. Since my improvement was really only true for lower body movements, however, another incarnation was in order.

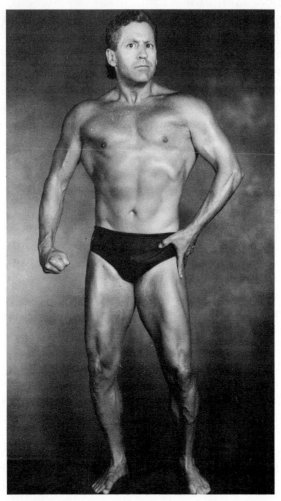

The author at forty-one when just starting again to specialize in bodybuilding.

Although there is some danger in copying verbatim another person's training program, I reasoned that no one knew more about training than Clarence. In addition, neither of us really could devote that much time to training because of our family and career responsibilities. Fortunately, we both enjoyed doing short (about one-hour), intense weight sessions (four per week) that focus around basic movements. Also, both of us have found that even shorter (30–40 minute) aerobic workouts (four per week), using variable equipment that complements body parts worked with weights on a given day, are very effective. Finally, we both enjoy walking on off-days (I no longer run). So, for me, Clarence's approach has proven to be a good match. I also follow most of Clarence's guidelines for optimal nutrition.

Within about six months on this schedule, I equalled or exceeded all the weights I had used in all exercises despite losing another five pounds. I equalled or exceeded not just totals from the year before, but *any* personal record (except one; see Chapter 4), even those made 20 years previously when I weighed 40 pounds more.

The results of this training schedule are detailed in Chapter 3 and are shown pictorially on the next page. Naturally, at this point, I started to think about masters competition and entered our state physique contest.

Initially I expected to win. The reality was that today competition at a state level and even at a masters level is extraordinary. I did not place.

However, seeing two excellent competitors in their 50s who placed ahead of me made me realize that I have a decade or more to *improve*. I now am focusing on how to slowly increase strength and gain some more mass while becoming much more muscular and defined.

At the same time, I am starting to feel the signs of a transition to yet another incarnation. Intense training has been enjoyable and rewarding, and I have surprised myself with how strong I can become on some movements, particularly using higher repetitions (see Chapter 3). If there were, for example, competitions on repetition squats with double body weight, I would be outstanding. Since there are not formal contests of that sort, it may be time to develop a new sport!

By training for the contest and improving my appearance

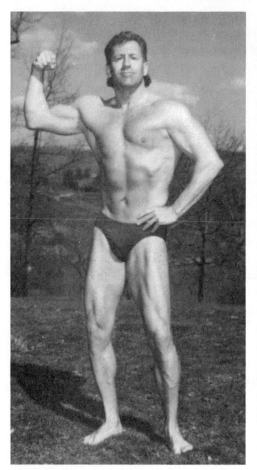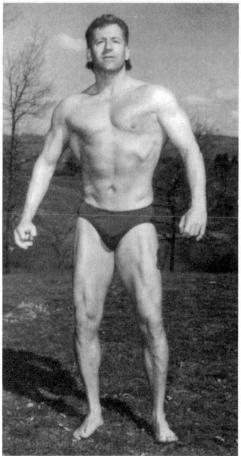

The author at forty-two after eight months on the periodization bodybuilding routine (see Chapter 3).

and strength, I proved a major point to myself. With intelligent and intense training, there is not necessarily an "inevitable decline" in physical performance, at least in early middle age. As my own case study, I had replicated some of Pollock's results.

Clearly, one purpose of a book for *Ageless Athletes* could be to describe an approach to intelligent and intense training. However, I also began to realize that my own research studies in psychology could form a major focus for a book.

Conceptualization Foundation and Focus

My original notion for this book was to place a major emphasis on theories of aging, attendant data, and the implications of that work for athletic training and performance in middle years. I still believe such an approach should be more fully developed, but I will only be touching on that topic in a later section of this book.

What became more apparent with a little reflection was that the most striking thing about masters athletes is that they display some extraordinary behaviors, usually over long periods of time. These people appeared to be super-motivated, if not all the time, at least most of the time.

Motivation and Behavior

Once I started to think more about motivation and behavior, several important and related ideas literally jumped at me. One of the biggest issues in psychology is "maintenance of behavior change." There are a number of principles, strategies, and techniques that are reasonably effective in helping people change initially, but when you look at the same people two, four, or six months after the initial, "successful" change effort, they are usually right back where they started—sometimes worse. Nowhere is this more the case than in trying to alter health-related behaviors such as smoking, weight control, and change in nutritional and exercise practices. In fact, there are now many studies in such areas (and with such unfortunate names) as "exercise compliance." Most of these studies have not shown great success either.

A Salutogenic Approach

In stark contrast to the results of these studies stands the example of the masters athletes. Many of these individuals hardly miss any workouts over many years. They are also usually quite rigorous with other health behaviors, such as diet. In other words, they show extraordinary persistence and motivation. While it is not fair to compare masters athletes doing their training and sports, say, to people struggling along in weight control and exercise programs (and, indeed, masters athletes may show a similar lack of motivation in other parts of their lives), it does make sense to me that a good deal may be learned about motivation and behavior by studying highly motivated individuals.

This approach is in contrast to considerable study in psychology, particularly clinical and health research, which has focused more on unmotivated individuals. This "pathological" emphasis can be questioned. For example, it has recently been demonstrated that many people have actually been successful on their own in stopping smoking or losing weight. The idea that these behaviors are incredibly difficult to change is based primarily on the poor outcomes of many clinical studies and projects, which have generally attracted less motivated and less successful individuals. In other words, an entire perspective with its supporting literature has been based on relatively select samples of unmotivated people.

In a similar way, the extensive literature on stress and coping has primarily focused on stress and psychological and physical breakdown. But, why not study those individuals who cope well with stress, who in some ways appear "invulnerable"? Indeed, for many years, Dr. Aaron Antonovsky has called for an almost total reorientation in the study of health behavior. His *salutogenic* model mainly emphasizes studying health-enhancing processes.

Overall, studying masters athletes could shed light on *motivation and behavior* and fit nicely with the emerging trend of studying healthful, adaptive processes.

Although I had not studied athletes and motivation, before most of the work I had done over my 16-year career focused on motivation and behavior. In the early part of my career, I set up programs in schools to help teachers become better instructors and to help children learn more quickly and proficiently. A long series of field studies in the middle part of my career revolved around strategies to motivate consumers to conserve energy (electricity, natural gas) in their homes. More recently, I have built on these earlier studies and focused on ways to motivate consumers to change health-related behaviors, such as nutritional practices.

Along the way, I had published many professional articles and received six major federal research grants, the last four from the highly competitive National Science Foundation and the National Cancer Institute. I had also developed a framework for designing and implementing motivational programs. I was considered an expert in motivation and behavior. Surely this expertise could be applied to athletic behavior and sports psychology.

A Sports Psychology Framework

As soon as I started to think along the lines of "sports psychology" and investigated some work in that area, a few other points also became apparent. The first was that much of that field was "technique driven." Different people were experts in particular strategies such as goal setting or mental training, but were really missing the larger picture. A coherent framework for understanding and modifying athletic behaviors was rarely evident. Virtually nothing that I saw or read represented the state of the art in psychology. It was true that athletes, coaches, and the general public thought that psychology could contribute a lot to sports, but what they were seeing so far was the proverbial "tip of the iceberg."

The kind of theory and framework that I used in many of my projects (and that a number of other researchers and practitioners used) had a great deal to offer the field of sports psychology and athletic training. Further, a good framework and its principles and strategies could integrate the various facets of athletic training and competition. For example, it does not make sense to have one theory and approach for physical training, another for mental training, and a third approach for competition. A good framework is adaptable to different behaviors and circumstances.

The Role of Studying Masters Athletes

At the same time, the study of exemplar individuals, even in a case study format, could not only help to verify aspects of a theory and framework, but perhaps could also help to expand

and modify the overall perspective and its elements. Frankly, as a psychologist, being able to contribute to conceptual development was both appealing and motivational.

The main way this task could be accomplished was through the study of a small sample of masters athletes. It seemed reasonable to study those individuals in sports that I had some experience with, namely endurance or strength sports. I quickly discovered through a few trial balloons that a number of masters endurance and strength athletes were not only accessible, but also eager to correspond and talk about their training and their lives in general. Their enthusiasm was contagious, and contrary to popular (and medical) belief, a number of these individuals reported that they were still improving. Their stories could be much more upbeat and optimistic than, for example, the older baseball player who was just hanging on.

The idea of doing "portraits" of exemplar masters athletes was sparked by Lloyd Kahn's *Over the Hill,* but I wanted to do a few things differently. I didn't want the portraits to be random in content; I wanted them to focus on long-term motivation and successful training and athletic behavior. While each of the portraits could be presented differently, they should all examine that theme.

In order to accomplish that task, a detailed questionnaire was developed. The questionnaire was either completed by the athlete, or extensive phone interviews were conducted, or both. Thus, there is some coherence to the portraits, and they form a mini, informal data base that expands upon the framework for this book.

So, a framework to study, understand, and improve upon athletic performance could form a basis for refining an already excellent approach (periodization) to training for different sports and for designing a comprehensive approach to mental training. The portraits could illustrate and expand upon the overall approach and strategies. And, then, I could pull all this information together and provide guidelines and principles for athletes of different aspirations and skill, with some of those guidelines adaptable to other parts of a person's life.

Retracing my steps in developing this book, then, I found through some study and personal experience that athletic performance could not only be stabilized in middle age, but also, in some instances, be improved. The study of masters athletes is personally fascinating and can also shed some light on important processes of long-term motivation and optimal performance to both illustrate and expand upon a psychological framework. This framework is one that encompasses and is adaptable to various facets of sports psychology. The overall perspective on training and motivation, and the principles and strategies of the framework, will help sophisticated masters athletes in their training, competition, and daily living. It is to the unfolding of the framework that we now turn.

2

A Systems Framework for Athletic Behavior and Motivation

Overview

A developing body of literature and research is starting to tell us a good deal about the physiology of masters athletes. Without a doubt, this biologically oriented approach will provide some excellent insights into the processes of aging, how these processes may be altered, and how alteration of the course of aging affects human performance in middle and older age. But, something very important is missing when following only this one perspective.

In the end, we may know much more about VO_2 max and strength levels of athletes through these studies than about what has *maintained the motivation and behavior* of these individuals whose VO_2 max and strength are off the charts. What sort of internal and external factors are at work here? What adjustments, if any, do these athletes make in their training to counter the effects of aging? How do these individuals set goals when performances of 10 years ago may no longer be obtainable? What types of cognitive ("mental") processes are effectively at work here? What types of personal beliefs are essential for athletic longevity? What kinds of support, feedback, and reinforcement do they receive from others? How do these athletes optimize reinforcement and other external influences? How do they fit training within hectic work and family schedules? How are reactions from other people changing as the middle-aged athlete becomes less of an oddball? And, as the middle-aged athlete becomes more the norm than the exception, has motivation for training been helped or hindered?

A Systems Approach to Studying Motivation

These questions imply that insights and answers about motivation require an approach that takes into account the interplays between internal and external factors. The word *interplays* means that each set of factors dynamically and reciprocally influences the other set of factors. *Dynamic* means that events and processes are constantly adjusting and changing. *Reciprocal influence* means mutual sets of influences. This simple schema is shown in Figure 1 and is the basic psychological foundation of this book.

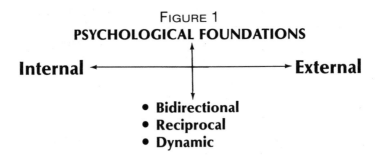

FIGURE 1
PSYCHOLOGICAL FOUNDATIONS

Internal ←————————————→ **External**

- **Bidirectional**
- **Reciprocal**
- **Dynamic**

The vertical bidirectional arrow (↕) implies change and movement. For example, people's fitness and their moods can vary a good deal, even in a short period of time. The horizontal bidirectional arrow (←→) means that one set of processes influences the second set which, in turn, influences the first set. For example, the internal standards of acceptable performance (e.g., to run two hard track workouts per week) that athletes set for themselves have a direct bearing on training and actual performance. The results of training and competitions generate feedback and reinforcement from other people, as well as self-evaluations and self-reinforcement, which may modify self-standards and, in turn, training and performance. These notions about dynamic and reciprocal processes and influences are basic elements of a *systems* approach. Thus, this book is probably the first to use a psychological systems approach to athletics.

Most applications of psychology to sports have been unduly simplistic and do not represent state-of-the-art concepts or perspectives. For example, many books, articles, and seminars only address the power of the mind and thought in athletics. Such an emphasis is important, but at best only represents part of the picture. Further, such nebulous terms as *will power* or *mental toughness* or *attitude* really tell us nothing. They are overused and general terms. Likewise, if we only focused on environmental factors such as reinforcement, we would also have a one-dimensional approach. People are neither automatons controlled by the environment, nor completely autonomous individuals thinking and behaving without influence and constraint. Indeed, even the word *motivation* is only a shorthand description (and inference) for various processes, influences, and behaviors. Although we will use the word *motivation* many times in this book, we must be aware that the word alone does not tell us much. Rather, to really understand motivation, we need to take a more sophisticated approach and focus on the interactions between individual thoughts, cognitive processes and techniques, behavior and performance, and specific environmental influences. These three sets of factors and domains (i.e., functions, processes, or influences)—cognition, behavior, and the environment—are also seen in a state of dynamic and reciprocal influence. This is shown in Figure 2.

FIGURE 2
BANDURA'S SOCIAL-COGNITIVE THEORY

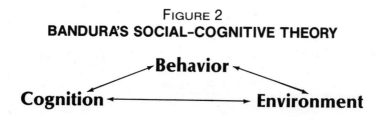

Just such a perspective and theory about cognition, the environment, and behavior has been developed by Dr. Albert Bandura of Stanford University. It is safe to say that Bandura's "social cognitive" approach is the dominant and most influential position today in psychology. This is undoubtedly true because his theory *integrates* internal and external processes (e.g., cognitions and environmental influences) and is *flexible,* constantly *evolving,* and very *useful.* For example, Bandura's theory, particularly those aspects related to motivation and behavior change, has been the basis of almost all the many community health promotion programs mounted in many different countries over the last decade. His approach also is a basis for probably the most widely used approach in psychotherapy, *cognitive behavior theory.*

The Impact of Feelings, Emotions, and Moods

For this book, I have adapted Bandura's approach—his overall perspective and research on specific processes and influences—and applied it to the special case of masters athletes. But I will expand upon Bandura's theory and principles. For example, it is important to add another important area—the affective domain of feelings, emotions, and moods—to Bandura's theory. Affective responses influence cognition, behavior, and the environment and can be very motivational. How we feel about our performance is of great importance. Figure 3, therefore, includes the affective domain in the theoretical schema.

FIGURE 3
BANDURA'S SOCIAL-COGNITIVE THEORY
(MODIFIED)

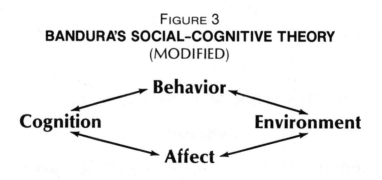

Hence, this book will offer a great deal to the study of athletes and optimal performance as well as to psychology. First, it provides a fresh approach to training and athletics. Second, it studies an exemplary set of individuals. As I noted in Chapter 1, all too often in psychology what we know about motivation and behavior is based on individuals who are unmotivated and display problems in at least part of their lives. In this book, we are studying competent people who show *extraordinary* motivation and performance in at least one part of their lives, athletics.

Specific Stages, Processes, and Influences

In the following sections of this chapter, I will describe specific cognitive, affective, behavioral, and environmental influences and processes. Although these influences and processes will be presented relatively discretely—in a vacuum, in a sense—it is important to always keep the notions of dynamic and reciprocal influence in mind.

It is also important to differentiate between different *stages* of motivation and behavior change. Bandura has described three stages: acquisition, generality, and sustained change. We will see these stages in action in Chapter 4, which provides a step-by-step approach to mental training. Here, the stages are only described.

When people are just beginning to become athletes or delve into a new kind of athletic activity, we can think of them as in a belief, behavior, and skill *acquisition* stage. For example, a few of the masters athletes featured in this book only became athletes in their middle years. Some of the processes and influences at this stage appear to be different from those that are important at later stages.

The next stage, *generality*, means that people display beliefs, behaviors, and skills under varying conditions. For example, when first taking up running (the acquisition stage), an athlete may only train with other supportive people, or with a coach giving constant encouragement and feedback, or only when the weather is good. In the generality stage, running will be done under many conditions—alone or with others, with or without a coach, in rain or shine.

In the *sustained* stage, beliefs, behaviors, and skills occur under various conditions for long periods of time—almost indefinitely. Some of the masters athletes featured in this book have been consistently training for 35 years! It is certainly this group of people who can tell us about motivation over the long haul. For these athletes in particular, we can see if how they think, feel, and behave *confirm* Bandura's theory and principles. At the same time, we should be able to *discover* processes and influences that enhance Bandura's perspective. This is because much of the research and writing in psychology on behavior change has only focused on the acquisition stage. Thus, this book can serve both functions: confirmation of existing theory and principles and discovery of new ideas and methods.

In addition, even the novice or nonathlete should find ideas and methods in this book that are applicable to optimal performance in athletics and other facets of life. For example, as we will see, many athletes are excellent at monitoring their performance in relationship to specific hard but reachable goals. This is a major and highly effective motivational strategy that can be used in acquisition, generality, or sustained stages by a wide variety of people for a wide range of purposes.

Cognitive and Affective Domains

Assuredly, people's beliefs, perceptions, thoughts, and feelings influence their behavior, and just as assuredly, behavior influences cognitive and affective processes. Three key cognitive processes will first be discussed: outcome expectancies, self-efficacy, and self-regulatory processes, particularly setting personal standards.

Outcome Expectancies

This term refers to beliefs that a specific course of action will lead to specific outcomes. In order to adhere to a rigorous training program, the athlete must believe that the program will yield certain desired results. For example, a runner believes that running three speed workouts per week in a specific way and order will lead to optimal speed increases for 10K races. Or, the athlete believes that following a very low-fat diet for three months will result in an optimal percentage of body fat and a lean, "ripped" appearance.

Outcome expectancies are "beliefs in the program." They are essential for success. That is why most athletes keep searching out the latest training information. And, perhaps, that's why some athletes are driven to try almost anything—drugs, fad diets, or all-day training.

A crisis occurs when, for any number of reasons, the athlete loses confidence in the effectiveness of the program. Moderate depression, anxiety, or even anger, are likely to result, and in the best case could lead to a search for more information, creation of a new program, renewed enthusiasm, increased confidence, and improved performance. In the worst case, clinically severe mood shifts may occur, and the athlete may become immobilized. Conversely, the athlete could overtrain, leading to injury and deepening his or her problems. This example of an initial loss of confidence in a program also nicely illustrates the interplays of cognitive, affective, and behavioral domains.

Self-Efficacy Belief

These beliefs are different from outcome expectancies. Self-efficacy is the athlete's belief that he or she is capable of a specific performance under specific conditions. Self-efficacy is *not* a general feeling or trait. These beliefs are *specific* to behavior, time, and place, and are absolutey essential for optimal performance.

A personal example can help differentiate self-efficacy beliefs from outcome expectations and show the critical role these beliefs play in training and performance. To do maximum-level high-repetition squats—15 repetitions—with a very heavy barbell—380 pounds—I must *believe* that I can do it.

That belief is self-efficacy. It is very specific. I probably would not believe that I could do 15 repetitions with 410 pounds under any set of conditions. And my beliefs about my squatting ability may have little relationship to my beliefs about bench pressing, much less to my beliefs about other parts of my life. The belief is not derived from thin air. It is based on careful training over time. For example, in two prior successive workouts, I may have squatted 15 times with 360 pounds and 15 times with 370 pounds.

It is obvious, then, that self-efficacy is the result of behavior, performance, and my *evaluation* of that performance. Self-efficacy beliefs can vary in strength and degree. For example, if I squatted 15 times with 370 pounds with ease, self-efficacy beliefs for 15 repetitions with 380 pounds will usually be very high. If it was a struggle to squat 15 times with 370 pounds, then self-efficacy beliefs for increasing to 380 pounds will usually be low, unless some other factor entered into the evaluation. If I had not warmed up well or had a slight cold and still did 15 squats with 370, I might believe that under more usual conditions, increasing to 380 would be a cinch.

These points (plus additional ones to be discussed shortly) yield the schema shown in Figure 4.

FIGURE 4
COGNITIVE PROCESSES

- Outcome Expectancies (Belief in the program)
- Self-Efficacy (Belief in own ability to perform a specific task)
- Self-Regulatory Processes

Beliefs ⟵⟶ Performance

Thus, self-efficacy beliefs set the stage for performance, and performance and evaluation usually result in more specific self-efficacy beliefs. This is one reason training programs that build in frequent attainment of successive goals are usually so effective. This point will be discussed further in Chapter 3 on periodization.

I can have optimal self-efficacy beliefs about my ability to do high-level squatting and at the same time have high, moderate, or even low outcome expectations. For example, I can believe that I can do the squat workout and reach my maximum leg size and strength. Or I may believe that while I can squat with the weight for the designated repetitions, my likelihood of achieving optimal outcomes is at best moderate or even poor. This may be because of my lack of belief in the program, overacknowledgment of genetic limitations, or perhaps devaluation of the outcome. For example, I may use Tom Platz or Chris Dickerson, two bodybuilders with probably the greatest legs of all time, as my yardstick for success. Whatever I would achieve would appear puny next to them.

It is apparent that optimal training and performance requires realistic and high self-efficacy beliefs and equally realistic and high outcome expectancies (see Figure 4). And, clearly, one set of beliefs can reciprocally influence the other set of beliefs positively or negatively. For example, as my self-efficacy beliefs about my squatting become more and more positive, it is likely under most conditions that my beliefs in the program will grow more positive. And, as my belief in the program continues, I am likely to approach my workouts with enthusiasm and confidence, resulting in better performance and more positive self-efficacy beliefs.

Self-efficacy beliefs and outcome expectancies explain one set of cognitive processes and the relationship of these processes to performance. But what keeps athletes "propelled" or striving to achieve high performance levels? For some athletes, it is obvious that extrinsic factors maintain high levels of performance. Some masters athletes continue to strive for trophies and adulation from other athletes and the public. And, of course, some (though not many) masters athletes make a good deal of money by training and competing. However, many masters athletes continue to follow rigorous training regimes in the absence of fame or fortune. And, clearly, some professional masters athletes are quite wealthy and ostensibly no longer need more prize money, however substantial that prize may be.

Personal Standards

The *personal standards* that individuals have set for themselves appear to be particularly critical in self-motivation processes. Standards can encompass consistency in training, performance in competitions, or appearance; indeed, any number of criteria. It is what the athlete holds dear that is important and motivating. Personal standards are also relatively specific to particular behaviors. This is not to say that standards cannot be broadened or changed. They can be modified by new information and self-analyses, performance evaluations, and feedback from others. However, the new standard can then become as motivating (or even more so) than the old standard.

Several key subprocesses help make self-standards regulatory and motivational. Once again, it is inappropriate to replace nebulous terms such as *will power* with *self-standards* and use the term as an explanation of the process and an outcome of the process (i.e., cause and effect). It is necessary to be more specific.

The key processes in setting self-standards involve self-observations, judgements of performance, self-reactions, and self-evaluations. Here, too, the processes are highly specific. Besides some fixed and central criteria of performance, such as distance and time run, weight lifted for a certain number of repetitions, points scored, and strikeouts, other dimensions of performance may be formally and informally noted and recorded. For example, athletes can note their degree of effort and concentration and the overall quality of their performance (e.g., their form in swimming). Self-observation occurs during the performance with immediate corrective functions, and it occurs after the performance, sometimes in fixed and sophisticated ways.

Self-Observation　　Formalized self-observation may consist of detailed records in a training log. Or, for some athletes, their every move is entered on a computer. This is often the case for every ball thrown by a major league pitcher. But even before the advent of computers as a day-to-day part of sports, pitchers such as Tom Seaver could recall in postgame interviews virtually *every* pitch they had thrown in a game, and the exact circumstances under which the pitch was thrown. For example, Seaver could identify the batter, the number of outs, the count, the men on base, and prior pitches to the same batter in the present and past games. Clearly, this is an example of sophisticated self-observation and remarkable recall ability.

Personal Judgement   Self-observations are typically subjected to personal judgements. Athletes will often assess how specific aspects of the performance compare to their personal standards. Was quality of the effort sufficient? Was concentration maintained throughout? How did the performance compare to their better prior efforts or to other athletes that they use as a yardstick? Can particularly good or bad performances be explained by external factors, resulting in a different interpretation of the performance? What is the overall personal evaluation of the effort?

Like self-observation, personal judgement can also be informal or highly formal. Some athletes have personal rating systems for their efforts using words or numbers. Some athletes discuss their evaluation of their performance with others as a way to formalize the process and receive feedback.

Self-Reaction   Self-Observations and judgements about performance result in self-reactions, that is, feelings, emotions, and mood states, which can be highly motivating. Meeting or exceeding standards, particularly when no other external factors contributed to a good or excellent performance, will usually result in very positive self-reactions. The athlete will usually feel good, sometimes exhilarated, and may develop self-rewards. These rewards for performance may consist only of self-statements ("You're really terrific!" "Great effort!"), or they may be more tangible. For example, the athlete may buy something special, go out for a special meal, or indulge in some favorite activities.

On the other hand, failing to meet standards, or meeting a standard only through external supports (being pushed by others, taking drugs, exceptional luck), is likely to lead to negative moods and self-punishment. Self-punishment can span the spectrum from negative self-statements, to self-censure and ridicule, to self-inflicted pain and deprivation.

Self-reactions, as noted, heavily contribute to an athlete's mood states and may, indeed, become *pervasive* mood states (e.g., depression) depending upon the importance for the athlete of the specific performance and the degree of meeting, exceeding, or failing to reach a self-standard. Self-judgements may, though, be very influenced by present mood states. For example, for a depressed athlete, a good, though not superior, performance may exacerbate depression. This, in turn, may lead to other less-than-ideal performances and further, deepening depression. These "spiralling" processes will be discussed later in this chapter.

On the brighter side, self-reactions are often highly motivating and lead to self-directed changes. The athlete who reaches or exceeds a performance goal and uses self-rewards often will be highly motivated to maintain or even improve upon already excellent performances. The athlete who falls short of self-standards but avoids a prolonged "funk" can become very analytical and use self-observations, judgements, and comparisons to improve performance. For example, the astute Tom Seaver was unlikely to make the same bad pitch to the same batter ever again. Or a runner may be sure never again to get caught up with the crowd, go out too fast, and tie-up at the end of a race.

Since many masters athletes are self-coached and not subject to very powerful external contingencies ("fame and fortune"), it must be concluded that *self-standard cognitive and affective processes are keys to athletic motivation.* Note, though, that these self-regulatory processes do not occur in a vacuum. They are highly dependent on behavior and environmental circumstances. Indeed, the regulatory processes influence performance in certain settings, and that performance is (self-) observed, judged, and reacted to—thus influencing subsequent performances. But where do personal self-standards come from?

Modeling   Quite often, and at least initially, personal standards reflect a *modeling* process. We learn through observing, reading, or hearing about other people. Modeling does not necessarily mean imitation, although it is not unusual for a beginning athlete to copy the demeanor and training regime of an "idol." Over time, through additional modeling experiences, corrective feedback, and comparisons to others, a self-standard is modified and often personalized. This seems particularly the case for masters athletes whose training and performance is in uncharted waters. For example, there has *never* been a top-level bodybuilder approaching 60 who looked like Bill Pearl or a track and field star like Al Oerter, now over 50 years old.

Nevertheless, we see in the development and modification of self-standards the interplay of cognitions, affect, and behaviors with the environment. Self-standards initially may be modeled from others. Over time with external feedback and self-feedback on performance—self-observations, judgements, and reactions—and additional modeling experiences, new self-standards evolve. These new self-standards may often provide an even greater degree of motivation since they have been fine-tuned by the tests of performance and feedback. All the key points about personal self-standards are summarized in Figure 5.

FIGURE 5
PERSONAL STANDARDS
(MATCH OR EXCEED)

- Self-Observations—Formal (logs), Informal—effort, quality, process (concentration)
- Judgments of Performance
- Self-Reactions (satisfaction, dissatisfaction; moods)
- Self-Evaluations (reinforcement, punishment) (self-statements, feedback)

Origins of Personal Standards

- Own
- Modeling
- Modify over Time

Athletic Behaviors

This section will discuss athletic behaviors, including those involved in training and recovery, competition preparation, competition, dietary selections, and use of drugs. When discussing training, it is easier to use as illustrations sports where training tends to be particularly systematized, such as running, swimming, and bodybuilding, as opposed to those that are more skill-based, such as gymnastics or golf, or where considerable conditioning is afforded through participation in a game such as basketball or hockey. Nevertheless, any sport does have a mix of skill acquisition, practice, and training (strength and endurance); and at higher levels, competition preparation and competition.

Training Variables

For training, the three key behavioral variables are frequency, duration ("volume"), and intensity. As with a range of other factors and influences already discussed, these three variables are interactive. Thus, the study of the training variables is also the study of a system. For example, very intense training usually must be done on a limited basis (frequency), for a limited amount of time (duration). Very frequent training will literally force the athlete to train at low levels of intensity. Training of very long duration places restrictions on frequency and intensity.

Regardless of the sport involved, athletes wittingly or unwittingly strike a balance between these variables. Often, that balance is a fragile one. Almost any alteration in a host of behaviors, or for that matter cognitive, affective, and environment influences, can upset the balance unless other *compensatory* changes are made. This point will be further illustrated at the end of this chapter.

It is widely agreed that improvement in endurance and strength sports only really comes from gradual and progressive *overloads*. In practice this means that at least occasionally the athlete must train very intensely. No amount of seven-minute miles can give the masters athlete aspiring to run a 4:50

mile the same effect as running interval sessions with repetition of 65–70-second quarter-miles. For the masters bodybuilder or lifter aiming for 10 repetitions in the squat with two-and-a-half times bodyweight, doing 50 repetitions with bodyweight will not help to fulfill that goal. Training effects are *specific*, and to reach high performance levels overloads must be judiciously and systematically applied, culminating in at least occasional intense training sessions. Much more is said about this topic in Chapter 3 on periodization.

In strength and endurance sports, the key training behavior is the ability to optimally perform in hard sessions. Everything else can be thought of as arranging and allowing that behavior to occur. It is in hard sessions and in competitions that all the other behaviors, feelings, cognitions, and environmental influences hopefully coalesce.

Unfortunately, one group of behaviors that sets the stage for such optimal training sessions and competitions has rarely been systematized. Athletes monitor, record, and (hopefully) creatively balance frequency, duration, and intensity. For example, for endurance sports, athletes are learning exactly what heart rates need to be achieved and sustained for improvement to occur. Similar study and ingenuity has generally been lacking for *recovery* behaviors.

Recovery

Recovery behaviors can be thought of as a continuum running from active to semiactive to passive recovery. Examples of active recovery include training at lower levels of intensity, performing alternate activities, also at low intensity levels, and stretching. A semiactive recovery may include planned meditation or relaxation sessions. Passive recovery includes sleep, rest, whirlpools, baths, saunas, and massage. The equation for recovery activities, including type, frequency, and duration necessary after intense training, at best remains intuitive and at worst is simply neglected.

Most athletes are quite adept at the training aspects of their sports. And, as you will see in the portraits, few masters athletes appear to require being pushed to train intensely. What most athletes need is to be as disciplined with recovery activities as with training. Indeed, it is probably the case that most serious athletes, regardless of age, would make new and sustained progress, *not* through acquiring a new training technique, but *by being more systematic with recovery.*

My own experience reflects on this point in both a positive and negative way. I have learned through repeated observations that regardless of activity (bodybuilding or aerobics), I make my best gains when my training sessions are relatively infrequent, short, but intense. I find intense, but brief, training enjoyable and productive. Also, because the volume is low, I recover better. However, this schedule still typically requires eight training sessions, four bodybuilding and four aerobic, per week. I do bodybuilding in the morning and aerobics in the late afternoon on the same days.

Many nonathletes have asked me how I fit all that training together with my family responsibilities and work schedule. They are often surprised with my response, which usually is: "The training sessions are short, so you just always schedule them in, like a meeting. That's not the problem. The problem is finding enough time for recovery."

Most likely in the future, many of the procedures such as feedback and goal setting used to enhance training performances will be creatively applied to recovery behaviors. At that point, new gains will be made by those athletes who follow the best approach to recovery.

Skills

Another set of behaviors that is more important for some sports than others is form and skill acquisition, and continued refinement, upgrading, and practice of those skills. For some sports, for example, distance running, skill acquisition is minimal, although even here frequent feedback on form can be invaluable. In other sports, such as gymnastics, most time and effort involves learning individual tricks or moves of increasing difficulty. They are used in sequences, "routines," for four different apparatuses, which are different for men and women. The innumerable tricks and increasingly difficult routines mean that compared to most other sports, the possible time involvement is virtually infinite. And, indeed, some gymnasts train all day, every day.

At the higher levels of such skill sports, since practice time so far exceeds that required in many other sports, many points in this book about balancing and scheduling other life pursuits become less relevant. Practicing a sport eight hours per day usually means there are not other life pursuits. Critical questions are whether such time is really required, and whether time has been simply expanded because it is possible to do so. For example, it is unclear how many times a move must be performed correctly in practice so that it can be performed perfectly in competition. Must the move be performed 20 times, 200 times, or 20,000 times? If successful study reveals that the answer is at the lower end, then dramatic time reductions could occur for skill sports. As gymnastics is presently practiced, it is not surprising that there are few adherents after the teenage years.

There are, however, a considerable number of masters athletes in sports where skill practice is a major component, such as tennis and golf. The critical acquisition requirements are exemplars of requisite skills, either through face-to-face, video, pictorial, or written instruction; practice time; and feedback. Time for practice and feedback are also required for skill upgrading and refinement. For masters athletes, a major problem is scheduling in sufficient time for skill practice.

Concentration

Skill acquisition and practice, and intense training and recovery, require other essential behaviors. For lack of better terms, the words *focused concentration* can be used. It is clear that without any specific training experiences, some individuals can bring all their thoughts, feelings, and behaviors to the task at hand. However, since many people have learned relaxation techniques, which can be a part of focused concentration, it seems likely that many people can be taught ways to better focus and concentrate (see Chapter 4).

The importance of these skills and abilities is widely acknowledged in diverse sports. For example, many top bodybuilders readily concede that superior genetics are most responsible for their outstanding appearance. However, they also note that a second major attribute is an extreme ability to concentrate during training. Perfectly executed exercises, with full extension and contraction, and deep mental concentration, they claim, can bring superior results even when only moderate weights are used. Likewise, the abilities to concentrate, closely self-monitor bodily responses, and subsequently alter form and effort have been noted as major skills of elite endurance athletes.

Expert instructions can demonstrate these skills for the athlete. Sustained practice may make them usable at will. It appears likely that the use of focused concentration skills can add much to any sports and training activities.

However, it is a mistake to believe that these skills only pertain to what is in the athlete's head. Assuredly, focused concentration works best with high self-efficacy beliefs and outcome expectancies. Is it possible to conceive of athletes effectively concentrating who do not believe strongly in their own abilities and who doubt the efficacy of their programs? However, other behaviors and circumstances, such as inadequate time for recovery and a stressful work schedule, can undermine the most fine-tuned beliefs and concentration abilities. As we have noted throughout this discussion, cognitions, affect, behaviors, and environmental influences are interactive. For optimal performance, all these factors must fit together.

Diet and Drugs

Other important athletic behaviors pertain to consumption: selecting food to obtain the best levels of calories and nutrients, and taking drugs, presumably to enhance training gains, performance, and recovery. Different sports have different beliefs and traditions with respect to diet and drugs. For example, bodybuilders have always believed that training was only part of the process. A good deal of muscle building was attributed to diet—exact proportions of nutrient and caloric intake.

In the not-too-distant past, bodybuilding was associated with often bizarre and unhealthy dietary practices. A typical bodybuilder's diet was high in protein and fat and low in carbohydrates. For the most part, this has been rectified. The contemporary bodybuilding diet is moderately high in protein and complex carbohydrates and very low in fat.

Throughout the 1960s and 1970s, the use of steroids in bodybuilding was rampant and, perhaps, still is. Uppers and relaxants were also frequently used. Recently, however, drug testing has been introduced prior to many contests, and the larger magazines in the field have taken an antidrug, prohealth stance. The exact results of these moves remain to be seen. One interesting by-product of the antidrug stance has been the proliferation of supplements to replace drugs, but these supplements are often of unknown effectiveness. In any case, the motives for the antidrug, prohealth position are mixed: protection of the sport's image on the one hand, profits for drug substitutions on the other hand.

Other sports have equally unfortunate histories. For example, because of their own self-imposed pressure and pressure from coaches and parents, female gymnasts often severely restrict calories, despite training for hours almost every day. Worse, studies with female gymnasts suggest that what they do eat often consists of "junk," high-fat and high-sodium snack food.

The common belief is that once the gymnast physically matures and gains weight, top-level competition days are over. This is partly true, but it is largely true because modern approaches to strength training (to compensate for weight gains) and sensible nutrition are infrequently incorporated into the training regime.

The drugs of choice for gymnasts tend to run more toward pain killers and anti-inflammatory drugs, probably because of the rigorous training and frequent minor injuries (through overtraining) involved in the sport.

Some sports, such as hockey and baseball, appear to have no particular tradition for dietary practices. Others, like tennis, are only now emphasizing nutrition. In contrast, a number of sports (e.g., football and basketball) have a rich history of the use of diverse drugs, while other sports (e.g., running) have frowned on the use of most drugs.

For many athletes in all sports, though, dietary practices have become important. To some degree, dietary changes reflect health consciousness raised by the mass media. However, most athletes will readily admit that if they do follow particular dietary practices, it is because they believe it will enhance performance and appearance. Bodybuilders, as noted, will often count every calorie and gram of protein and fat. Runners will gorge themselves for several days before long races with every possible carbohydrate within reach. Gymnasts will deliberately not eat.

Likewise, the major reason that athletes take drugs is the belief that they will improve performance. The drug will help the athlete grow, or aid recovery, or mask pain, or fine-tune alertness. Thus, athletes turn to diet and drugs because of high outcome expectancies. Recall that one meaning of this term is "confidence in the program."

If the program is followed with real or imagined positive results, outcome expectancies are increased. Likewise, other cognitive changes may occur, but the kind and degree of change is difficult to predict. Self-efficacy beliefs concerning the ability to train hard and perform excellently may be increased. But these beliefs may have an important *qualification* related to the causal attributions. The athlete may often believe that: "I know I can do great at that competition if I continue to take that drug." Such a combination of cognitions and beliefs is likely to lead to sustained drug use.

Thus, dietary and drug practices, which for some athletes obsessively take center stage, again illustrate the interplay of cognitions and behaviors. Likewise, as we will see later, these behaviors also point toward what will be called "macro" (e.g., mass media) and "micro" (e.g., modeling of drug use by other athletes) environmental influences.

Competition

Peaking   Preparation for competition and actual competition intensifies all the behaviors that have been noted. Training must become harder, diets must be more rigorously followed, and heightened vigilance and concentration must be maintained. These practices are generally referred to as *peaking*. The peaking process differs between sports. At one extreme, many bodybuilders usually peak for only one or two contests per year, and often these contests will be close in time. This is peaking for the moment. Indeed, one of the all-time greats in bodybuilding told me that he became so proficient at the peaking process that he could reach his peak for the year at the exact time during the day of competition when it was necessary to look his absolute best.

At the other extreme, a major league baseball player in a tight pennant race and playoffs, where every game is a "must win," may have to maintain close to peak performance every day for two months. This is a challenge of another sort.

The term *peaking* does, however, imply that the condition is special and relatively short-lived. There is a long and gradually intensified buildup to high levels of performance, and then there is an inevitable decline. Peaking is difficult for professional athletes, and usually more so for the amateur. That is because it requires that "all systems are go." The athlete is vulnerable and is often running a fine line between improvement and injury, or even collapse. Any training error, environmental intrusion, negative mood, or doubt in oneself or the program can be a disaster.

Also, many athletes forget that intensification of training and other related behaviors requires much more attention to recovery. This is also where the amateur suffers. It is difficult to find the time for more rest, sleep, or other restorative activities. Bill Rogers, now a masters athlete, has said for many years that people working full time could not compete with him because they cannot find the time for proper recovery.

However, the periodization approach to be described in Chapter 3 is a method to systematically achieve peaking, primarily through controlling training stress and recovery. It is most appropriately used by athletes who can gear up for only major competitions during a year, although in principle the approach is useful for all athletes.

For many athletes, after sustained training and the rigors of peaking, competition may be the easiest part. This may be particularly true since prior to competition many athletes go through a brief (about a week) tapering phase in which they reduce the volume and intensity of training. In any case, competition presents the opportunity for valued tangible, social, and personal rewards that result when exceptional abilities have been honed over a long period of time.

Focused Concentration   Numerous writers and athletes have noted that a requisite for success in competition is a state of relaxed vigilance and confidence. I have called it *focused concentration*. Others have referred to the state as "being in the zone." It can mean an extraordinary ability to pick up the rotation on a 95-mile-per-hour fastball, or the equally extraordinary ability to run most of a marathon just below an anaerobic threshold by constantly self-monitoring effort and feelings and making adjustments.

Obviously, terms are not valuable in themselves, and it is not valuable to give the terms a magical aura. What is valuable is to be able to functionally describe the cognitive and behavioral skills and environmental supports that are required so that athletes can practice them to perfection. More will be said about this topic in Chapter 4.

Longevity   It is also apparent that longevity in a sport is related to success—the outcomes that are achieved—but here one major caveat must be introduced. In reality, of course, few people achieve a high level of success in any sport. By definition, there are few champions, "number ones," among many participants. If success as typically defined in our society—winning—was the key to longevity, then there would be very few masters athletes. This suggests that other definitions of success and effectiveness are needed, and that many masters athletes have found such definitions.

Perhaps one inkling of what is most important psychologically for longevity is found by looking at athletes who were successful, who "won," in their teens, 20s, or 30s, and by their early middle years appear hopelessly sedentary, unfit, and overweight. The masters athlete has a hard time understanding such people, since these athletes were so gifted when younger and very little would have been required to maintain some semblance of fitness.

It is possible that such formerly great athletes were mainly motivated by the final rewards of winning: fame and fortune. This point is not meant to demean such aspirations and extraordinary efforts. It is difficult to fault the youngster who makes it out of poverty through boxing or a track scholarship. But once the glory days are over, what replaces fame and fortune (or the real fear of poverty) as a motivator? It is also quite possible that many athletes who do not continue at least fitness activities after their competitive days simply never really *enjoyed* the training and attendant activities. In fact, training may have been extremely painful. It was only a means to an end.

In contrast, longevity in athletes seems to require an enjoyment of the process. Not every workout is great fun, and putting together a training schedule with family and work responsibilities is not an easy task. Yet, overall, there must be a general liking of the activities, a continued sense of confidence in oneself and the program, the challenge of striving to meet goals, the satisfaction of meeting some personal standards, and reasonable environmental supports. This is another definition of success.

For longevity, cognitive, emotional, behavioral, and environmental factors must fit together, and the athlete must genuinely like the means—the athletic behaviors. In fact, in this analysis, the end, the major goal, is to continue the means.

Environmental Influences

Self-standards and the attendant self-regulatory processes are keys to sustained motivation and athletic behaviors. However, thoughts, feelings, and behaviors occur in, and are influenced by, environmental circumstances. As we have noted, this is a reciprocal process so that thoughts, feelings, and behaviors that were influenced by the environment, in turn, will influence environmental circumstances for particular athletes.

Reinforcement and Feedback

Probably every reader knows that rewards, or as we psychologists say, "reinforcements," following behaviors serve to maintain or increase those behaviors, and negative outcomes, or punishments, following behaviors tend to decrease or eliminate those behaviors. However, this is hardly a mechanical, fixed process, and it is a mistake to think about reinforcement and punishment in that way.

Reinforcement or punishment need not always be very immediate, as once thought, to be effective. In fact, *anticipating* future reinforcers is very motivating for many athletes. Hence, we see athletes training at a high level for many months for a future competition. And, often, the reinforcer for many masters athletes may not be winning the competition but simply being able to "be there."

Thus, reinforcers or punishers are not necessarily tangible, like money or even trophies. Rather, most people are particularly affected by positive social reinforcement, such as praise from others, and negative social reinforcement such as verbal disapproval, or nonverbal signs (e.g., frowns) from people the athlete values (e.g., fellow athletes, coaches). We can call these positive and negative sources of environmental influence *feedback*. Feedback provides information about our effectiveness in the environment related to some objective or purpose.

However, people do not respond as a simple robot would to information input. First, people's perception of their environment colors what they see, a point that we will return to later. Secondly, people actively evaluate information—its source, intensity, credibility, and usability. Based on that evaluation, they may or may not alter their response. For example, with feedback from a valued swimming coach on form, the performance of particular strokes is likely to be altered. However, the swimmer could ignore the feedback or integrate the feedback with other information and modify strokes in a unique way. In addition, people can alter the nature of the feedback by seeking out feedback from other coaches or knowledgeable swimmers or having themselves videotaped and providing their own feedback. Again, it is helpful to view people *not* as autonomous from their environments, but rather as partial architects of their environments.

Self-generated feedback *can* be very motivational, particularly when feedback has a relationship to specific, hard, but reachable *goals*. Feedback in the absence of specific goals is *not* very effective. Likewise, a specific goal without frequent feedback is also not very effective for motivating behavior. The two go together.

In Chapter 3 on training, *periodization* will be discussed as it applies to a number of different types of athletic training. Besides its physiological virtues, periodization appears to be so effective because of the specificity of goals, immediacy of feedback, and the overwhelmingly positive nature of the feedback.

For appropriately developed training systems, we are aiming for immediate, positive feedback. This is an old, but true, notion from psychology about the importance of immediate, positive reinforcement for maintaining motivation and behavior on a day-to-day basis. People do not necessarily need constant, specific feedback and goals, but it does help!

Note also how the external processes involved in feedback and goal setting fit with the internal processes of self-observation, self-judgements, self-incentives, and self-standards. For example, in my training log, a specific goal weight and number of repetitions is designated for every exercise for every session. The weights and repetitions come from considerable self-analysis and planning, and depend upon the immediately prior training sessions and the training cycle. Making the specified repetitions for a given weight in an exercise is highly satisfying to me, particularly so for sessions in the last stage of a training cycle. Successful execution leads to certain observations and judgements about myself, for example whether or not the repetitions were easy and made in good form. These observations and judgements result in particular feelings and a sense of fulfillment or nonfulfillment of my personal self-standard. Particularly good or poor feedback often leads to attempts to alter a subsequent round of feedback. For example, with poor feedback—failure to meet goals—I seek out the advice of people knowledgeable about bodybuilding and try to modify my training. With good feedback—meeting and exceeding goals—I readily admit that I like to tell people about my success. The enthusiasm and congratulations received from knowledgeable others can often provide training inspiration for many months, resulting in strict adherence to my schedule and the ability to surpass new goals.

Again, it is important to understand the specific reinforcement techniques and processes and the interactivity between people and their environments. People do not completely control their environments, and their environments do not completely control them. Reciprocity is at work. However, the point is that *athletes have it within their abilities to hook themselves into powerful feedback systems* which can help them maintain high levels of motivation. The feedback can come from people, training logs, or any other meaningful source of information. There are, however, other important environmental influences that need to be examined.

Modeling

As suggested before, *modeling* is a very effective way to change behavior. Although modeling is not imitation, it is a process where information about behavior is provided through observation, reading, or word-of-mouth with little need for extensive trial and error. We can take what we feel are the best and most appropriate aspects of an exemplar athlete's training system and apply it to ourselves.

Models are more likely to be emulated if their behaviors are valued and reinforced and if the model's characteristics bear some approximation to the observer's characteristics (real or hoped for). Thus, a few exemplar masters athletes can have a great impact. They are likely to inspire some individuals who probably will become models for others. Modeling is at the heart of what has been called the "diffusion of innovations," the spreading of new ideas and behaviors. In the case we are discussing, the innovation is the beliefs, thoughts, and behaviors about being athletic in the middle years.

In addition, the exemplar athlete can become an important molder of self-standards, and such standards, as we have seen, are central to long-term motivation. Successful modeling of another individual will also, hopefully, result in considerable external reinforcement.

Thus, the athlete has a personal environment and a more general environment that includes models, feedback, and reinforcement.

In the last 15 years, the number of masters athletes has greatly increased, and not surprisingly, so has the social acceptability of engaging in athletics in the middle years and beyond. In the early 1970s, the 44-year-old runner would have been hard-pressed to find many known, top middle-aged runners to emulate. The most likely reactions from other people to the 44-year-old runner then were bewilderment, warnings, and scorn. Training was most often done alone, and masters races were few and far between.

Today, the 44-year-old runner can find many near-age models, supportive reactions from many people, and numerous clubs and races. And the novice 42-year-old bodybuilder today can choose among a number of different gyms, even in a small town. She may be following the advice and routines of the middle-aged and phenomenal Kay Baxter, and may even find her co-workers urging her to enter her first contest. Her immediate supervisor at work may also be willing to allow her to follow a more flexible work schedule so she can better balance her family, training, and work responsibilities.

Macro and Micro Influences

These briefly made points remind us that modeling, feedback, and reinforcement processes depend upon a supportive context. Such macro-level influences as economics (which can provide for or limit athletic pursuits), mass media portrayals of middle-aged athletes, and evolving social beliefs and norms about aging and athletics do have direct effects on thoughts, feelings, behaviors, and environments pertinent to athletics. We can also see that there is a reciprocal influence between macro influences and personal processes and environments. For example, money provided by corporate sponsors provides the impetus for top-rung and middle-of-the-pack runners to train harder and compete in newly available races. Subsequent large turnouts and media attention given to the participants and races will often result in more corporate sponsorship and more races.

Macro-level influences are inevitably important in examining the behavior and motivation of individuals and groups. At times, they will be part of the discussion in this book. However, as a psychologist, I am more comfortable examining the role of micro-environmental influences and issues such as social support from others, access to settings, and control of schedules. Inclusion of these environmental factors still provides a more expansive approach to motivation than is generally offered from sports psychology. And, it is in the social and setting realms that individual processes of motivation are played out, with such influences greatly facilitating or hindering individual initiatives. We will now discuss these influences in some detail.

Some individuals may appear to be unmotivated for athletic and fitness activities. Or, conversely, other people may appear to be trying very hard to succeed but getting nowhere. In these instances, it is easy to blame the athletes for their shortcomings. Extensive, but often misguided, analyses of persons' strengths and weaknesses may be conducted. However, from the top athlete to the fitness buff, *the best starting point for an analysis of motivation is an analysis of the environment.*

As noted before, a number of influences should be part of environmental analyses, including:

- *Social Supports.* What kinds of encouragement and support are available and frequently given by other people or organizations? And, what kinds of negative feedback from others are given for athletic pursuits? What effects do these social influences have on the athlete, and how can they be altered to maximize performance?

- *Setting Factors.* What settings are necessary and available for training? What obstacles preclude ready or easy access and use? Do these settings facilitate or hinder performance?
- *Schedule.* What is the athlete's training schedule? How do the times and places for training fit with family and work responsibilities? Does the schedule allow for optimal performance in different parts of a person's life?
- *Training Regime.* What exactly is the regime, its frequency, intensity, and duration? In particular, how does the regime fit with setting and schedule factors? Is there ample time for quality efforts, and just as important (if not more so), is there ample time for recovery?

Motivation and Environments

Clearly, other environmental factors such as diet and weather conditions can be considered as part of this mix of factors. The most basic point, however, is that while individual cognitions, affect, and behavior may overcome some hindering environmental influences, it is quite apparent that *the best mix of factors for maximizing performance entails optimizing individual initiative and environmental influences.*

It is also necessary to recall the basic notions of reciprocity. For example, highly motivated athletes will often seek to maximally arrange their environment to facilitate training and performance. Because the environment is so arranged, optimal efforts are possible, bringing optimal results, thus maximizing motivation. Clearly, here we see the interplay of cognitive, affective, behavioral, and environmental factors. And, indeed, the example also suggests an important *upward spiralling ef-*

fect. As one set of factors is maximized, for example, efficacy beliefs and personal standards, the effect is to maximize another set of factors, such as the training schedule, which feeds back and increases the first set, and so on. This effect is illustrated in Figure 6.

We can also briefly examine what results when, for example, environmental factors are not carefully considered. This often happens when people are just starting fitness programs or when athletes must take on new responsibilities in different parts of their lives. Training is disrupted or best efforts yield minimum returns. In the worst case, the athlete feels and performs more and more poorly. Environmental hindrances and subpar performance undermine individual motivation. Indeed, here it is easily possible to predict a *downward spiralling effect.* This effect is also shown in Figure 6.

FIGURE 6
High Level Performance = High Motivation =
Optimizing Individual Initiative &
Environmental Influences

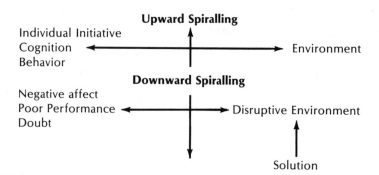

All too often under these circumstances, and this is most often the case with dedicated athletes, they will try harder and harder. The typical result is frustration, depression, doubt, and highly diminished self-efficacy beliefs and outcome expectancies. Injury or other physical breakdowns are likely. The solution to this dilemma does not lie on the individual side of the equation. It resides on the environmental side. Settings and schedules need to be altered. When this is not possible, training variables (e.g., frequency) and goals need to be adjusted.

There are, however, instances where attention to the individual side of the equation does make a good deal of sense. Sometimes environmental factors are or could be relatively optimal, but the athlete *perceives* that they are far from ideal. In the first instance, there may be a substantial difference between subjective and objective reality. In the second instance, the environment may be modified and controlled, perhaps by rearranging work and training schedules, but the athlete perceives that there is no control. Perceived inability to control the environment has often been linked to stress and depression, at times to a clinically severe degree.

Changing faulty beliefs requires that a coach, friends, or fellow athletes point out inconsistencies between the athlete's thoughts and objective reality. For example, an athlete who feels that his hard training efforts are not acknowledged by others (when in reality they are) can be asked to recall positive feedback statements from others. An athlete who feels that her environment has become uncontrollable (when, in fact, it can be dealt with) can be given a simple step-by-step approach to control, for example, through time management strategies (see Chapter 4 for a general approach to a process of behavior change).

Hopefully, these points about perceiving the environment will not lead to the conclusion that motivational problems are always "head cases." Rather, the contention is still that any approach to maximizing motivation should start with an environmental analysis.

And, hopefully, in a more general way, the extended discussion in this chapter shows that motivation is not just a simple matter of willpower or mind over matter. To understand both short-term and long-term motivation, we are always interested in the interplay of cognitions, affect, behavior, and the environment.

THE OVERALL FRAMEWORK

Figure 7 (page 52) summarizes the different cognitive, environmental, and behavioral influences and processes related to optimal athletic performance. It is not a neat or one-dimensional framework. This chapter has discussed the interplay of many different kinds of factors and has repeatedly warned about simplistic explanations of human behavior.

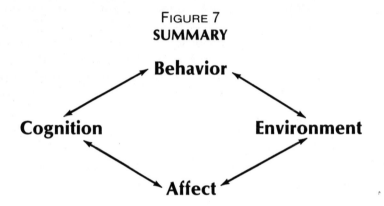

FIGURE 7
SUMMARY

Maximize
- Cognitions and Affect
- Outcome Expectancies
- Self-Efficacy
  - Self-Regulatory Processes
  - Self-Observations
  - Self-Evaluations
  - Self-Reactions (Enjoyment, Satisfaction)
- Behavior
  - Optimal Mix of Frequency, Intensity, Duration
  - Stress/Recovery
  - Build-up   Peak-Tapering
- Environment
  - Feedback/Goals
  - Modelling
  - Support, Settings, Schedule, Regime

When confronted with such a framework, its complexity and the many possible interactions that it suggests and that have been discussed, can be overwhelming. For an approach to have any value over and above being an interesting intellectual exercise, it must be useful. This framework has much greater utility for the individual athlete, coach, trainer, or educator, than simpler approaches. This is because the framework suggests *many pathways for change that can have reverberating and spiralling effects.*

Utility

For example, let's take the case of an athlete who is having difficulty balancing family, work, and training responsibilities. As one solution, more flexible hours are arranged at work—an environmental change. One immediate effect is an increase in self-efficacy beliefs about having optimal workouts. Because of these beliefs and the schedule change, workouts indeed can be performed more intensely. Others notice the better workouts and provide the athlete with support and praise, and the feedback from a coach is quite positive. The athlete meets or exceeds certain goals that the coach has set, as well as her own personal standards. She is extremely happy and verbally and tangibly reinforces herself. She has much greater confidence in the program (outcome expectancies). Her self-efficacy beliefs are further increased. The athlete now puts even more effort into her workouts. This process, which started with one simple but strategic change, has had reverberating and upward spiralling effects.

Another example involves an athlete who is frequently tired, has some minor injuries, is stuck at a plateau of performance, is becoming depressed, and is beginning to experience some sleep disturbances. These are classic symptoms of overtraining. The wise athlete or coach, recognizing these symptoms, would first make changes on the behavioral side. For example, the number of training sessions could be slightly reduced and greater rest and sleep prescribed.

A likely result is that better recovery occurs, leading to more intense training, more positive feedback and support from others, goal attainment, more positive self-efficacy beliefs, self-reinforcement, more positive outcome expectancies, and harder workouts.

Thus, if the initial assessment of the problem is reasonably correct, it can be expected that the change will have multiple and probably synergistic effects.

These last two examples of change are shown in Figure 8. They present a highly positive, though not a Pollyanna, approach to change and optimizing performance.

FIGURE 8
EXAMPLE OF PATHWAYS FOR CHANGE WITH REVERBERATING AND SPIRALLING EFFECTS

Modify the Environment

Modify work schedule to allow more control and rest and recovery

- Increased Self Efficacy
- Increased Performance and Gains
- Better Feedback and Social Support
- Reach Goals
- Exceed Standards
- Self Reinforcement
- Greater Outcome Expectancy

Modify a Behavior

Modify training schedule (Overtraining: Decrease Frequency, Maintain Intensity and Duration; More Rest)

- Greater Ability to Train Intensely
- More Positive Feedback and Support
- Goal Attainment
- Higher Self Efficacy
- Self Reinforcement
- Higher Outcome Expectancy

Summary

Athletic training, high-level performance, and long-term motivation reflect an interplay of cognitive, affective, behavioral, and environmental influences. These influences and processes can be enumerated and defined. Each set of factors is best seen as in a dynamic state of reciprocal influence. Although this systems framework is by no means a simple one, it offers a more complete way to study and understand athletic behavior and motivation. And, most importantly, the framework provides for many avenues to alter and enhance motivation and performance.

In the next chapter, we will see how these same principles form the cornerstone for a markedly effective training system.

3
Periodization: Optimizing Training and Psychological Principles

The best training system and complementary routines will be detailed in this chapter. The system is called periodization. It is applicable to a variety of training endeavors and sports, and is an approach that fits nicely with the psychological principles described in Chapter 2. One word of caution—if you closely follow periodization principles, you will likely succeed beyond your wildest expectation!

Most of my experience with periodization is in bodybuilding and various aerobic activities. As I noted in the introductory chapter of this book, Clarence Bass, a former over-40 Mr. America, gave me a blueprint for periodization at about the same time that I started to emphasize bodybuilding and deemphasize running. I cannot attribute all the gains I made in a comparatively short time to periodization, but I feel a good part of my progress was, and continues to be, the result of using this system.

Table 1 shows what periodization did for me:

TABLE 1

Date: September 1985			Date: April 1987		
Exercise	**Wt.**	**Reps**	**Exercise**	**Wt.**	**Reps**
Bench Press	180	8	Bench Press	215	8
Squat	300	8	Squat	410	8
Stiff/Leg Dead Lift	285	8	Stiff Leg/Dead Lift	315	15
Dip	80	8	Dip	105	8
Leg Press	600	15	Leg Press	730	15
Curl	100	8	Curl	125	8
Dumbbell Sidebend	100	8	Dumbbell Sidebend	135	8

Measurements		**Measurements**	
Weight	162 lbs.	Weight	152 lbs.
Chest	45"	Chest	47.5"
Waist	31"	Waist	28.0"

There are a number of important points about the strength gains. Although I am stronger in my lower body, the gains were reasonably proportional across movements and body parts, and over the eighteen months. As I made these gains, I was reducing my body weight, and of course, I was getting older. Finally, I was reasonably strong at the start, not a rank beginner. Thus, I can attest from experience—periodization really works!

THE SYSTEM

Periodization, a system developed in the Soviet Union by Dmitri Matveyev, closely follows Hans Selye's classic response to stress syndrome, but with several differences. Readers will recall that Selye described three stages in response to stress—alarm, resistance, and exhaustion. Periodization is designed to modulate alarm, control the process of resistance and adaption, and *avoid* exhaustion and breakdown. In other words, periodization provides superior control over stress and recovery cycles. You gradually enhance performance and experience few, if any, breakdowns and injuries.

The origins of periodization can be traced back about 50 years. As athletes began to train year 'round for specific sports, it became apparent that no one could train hard month after month. At first, training intensities and modalities were fitted around the seasons of the year. In some sports, especially those where competitions cluster at particular points, this approach still makes sense. Thus, a track person who wants to peak for summer events could do background, base work in the winter, sharpening in the spring, racing in the summer, and recovery training in the fall. However, even with these circumstances, training can be more systematic, varied, and productive if periodization is followed. For example, seasonal phases for training include cycles that are too long and relatively unvaried.

Periodization Cycles

Periodization typically involves short cycles that vary the intensity and volume of training. Drs. Michael Stone and Harold O'Bryant, probably the two individuals who have best articulated and researched periodization, refer to a short cycle of about four weeks as a *micro-cycle*. A *meso-cycle* generally contains three micro-cycles, and a *macro-cycle* can represent a whole year of several meso-cycles. However, it is also possible to think of macro-cycles as covering longer time frames, for example, a four-year build-up to the Olympics.

Across three micro-cycles, intensity is gradually increased while volume is gradually decreased. This means that a meso-cycle always starts with easier, low-intensity, high-volume workloads and ends with much harder, high-intensity, but much lower volume workloads. Thus, a peak is reached. After the peak, there is a one- to two-week active rest phase, and then the procedure starts again but at a slightly higher level. ("Active rest" means engaging in low-intensity sports—such as easy walking, swimming, or noncompetitive sports—and usually these activities are not related to the athlete's primary sport.)

A prominent feature of the system is that every workout has

specific goals that are almost always achieved although they become successively harder. Thus, psychologically, the grounds for success are very fertile, a point to be discussed later in this chapter.

An Illustration of Periodization

Figure 1 is based on an adaption of Stone and O'Bryant's work, as well as Bass's application of periodization to bodybuilding. To illustrate how periodization works, only one exercise, the squat, has been chosen. This is admittedly an idealized, though not impossible to achieve, meso-cycle.

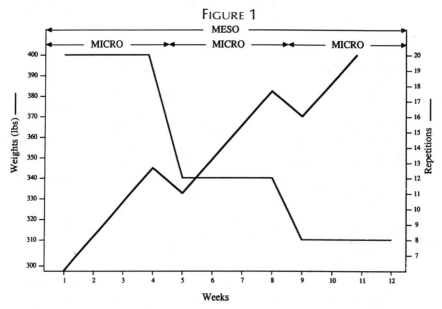

FIGURE 1

The volume of the workload is primarily represented by the repetitions (right side of figure), while the intensity mostly involves the weight (left side of figure). The meso-cycle, as shown on the figure, starts with high repetitions (20) and low intensity (300 pounds), but ends with lower repetitions (8) and high intensity (400 pounds).

Each week's weight for the squat (and here, it is assumed

that there is only one hard workout per week per movement) has been predetermined. It is a reachable, *progressive* goal, each week. Usually, a weight will be increased by several percent each week. Usually, a weight will be increased about 5 percent in the beginning of a micro-cycle, but only about 3 percent at the end of the cycle.

The athlete who follows periodization meets each weight and repetition goal. Often, each micro-cycle ends in a personal record for the weight and repetition scheme. The start of each micro-cycle, however, is easy. This is an extremely critical point that makes the whole system work. For example, note on the figure that even though the second and third micro-cycle lower the repetitions (12 and 8, respectively) and hence the volume, the weight is still *decreased* a few percent to start a new micro-cycle. This is because the end of a micro-cycle requires more intense, difficult training, which is both physically and psychologically taxing. Consequently, these efforts make greater inroads in recovery and overall training enthusiasm. It makes sense that the next week may be a bit flat and require lower intensity.

There is another reason for starting quite easily in a micro-cycle. The idea is to always be successful and by starting easier, you assure this result. You also get a breather so you can really build physically and emotionally through the next micro-cycle.

Although this section has used weight training as the activity to illustrate how periodization works, it should be apparent that different kinds of training can readily fit within periodization. For example, with running, the first phase would focus on longer, slower runs. The second phase would have moderate distance and moderate speed, and the third phase would be geared toward shorter distances and speed.

Interval Training and Periodization

An excellent way to do all kinds of aerobics is through interval training. Interval training entails bursts of higher intensity activity—"repetitions"—interspersed with timed periods of lower activity or rest—"intervals." The repetitions are at a more intense level than can be sustained for a long period of time. Thus, it is believed that interval training is one way to receive a high-level training stimulus without exhaustion.

It is easy to see how well interval training fits with periodization. The first micro-cycle features training sessions with a relatively large number of easy to moderate intensity repetitions for a longer duration. The second micro-cycle reduces the number of repetitions and their duration but shifts up to moderate intensity. The last micro-cycle, of course, has only a minimal number of repetitions of short duration but of high intensity.

PARTICULARS OF THE MICRO-CYCLES

Different people in the field have used different names for micro-cycles and, in some ways, have ascribed different functions to them. For example, Michael Stone and Harold O'Bryant are more oriented to strength training—weightlifting and powerlifting for competition or for strength athletes. Jan and Terry Todd have adopted the Stone and O'Bryant system for conventional weight training. Not surprisingly, the creative Clarence Bass has taken the system several steps further.

The Stone and O'Bryant System

The Stone and O'Bryant system has the phases shown in Table 2:

TABLE 2

Phase	Time	Sets	Repetitions	Volume	Intensity
Hypertrophy	4 weeks	3–5	10	High	Low
Basic Strength	4 weeks	3–5	5*	Moderate	Moderate
Power	2 weeks	3–5	2–3*	Low	High
Rejuvenation	1–2 weeks	vary	vary	Low	Low

*can include one back-off set of 10 repetitions

Note that during the Basic Strength and Power Phases, a back-off set of ten reps for each exercise may be included. This is because Stone and O'Bryant have found that with lower repetitions there is some loss of muscle mass and an increase in percent of body fat. While this system has been shown to work with a wide variety of athletes in a number of sports, their specific blueprint is *not* recommended for two reasons:

1. Doing the same exercise for many sets can be boring and not that productive.
2. The low repetitions of the Basic Strength and Power Phases now are felt by a number of athletes and coaches to be dangerous and counterproductive.

Whatever benefits are gained from the very low repetitions are outweighed by the costs. Further, for most people, training in the low repetition range presents the same problems and tradeoffs as for the strength athletes.

Bass and Exercise Physiology

Bass's adaption of periodization can work for any person regardless of age, sex, or experience in training. Besides the notion of phases, Bass also incorporated some of the ideas of Fred Hatfield (a champion power lifter, an exercise physiologist, and former editor for Weider publications) into his system. Hatfield has postulated that each component of a cell performs a specific function and that, therefore, each component must be stressed in a different way in order to effectively achieve overload.

In simplistic terms, the *myofibrils* are the strength component of the cell, while the *mitochondria* are the endurance part. It is thought that relatively explosive repetitions of weight-training exercises in the 6–10 range best affect the myofibrils, while slow repetitions in the 15–25 range affect the mitochondria component. Moderately performed mid-range repetitions, 10–15, may affect both components.

I think the proper word used above is *may*. Debates continue in exercise physiology about the specificity of training and cellular response. I do not claim to have the answers. I do know from experience that by systematically varying the repetition range and performance of an exercise, I get a welcome change in the training stimulus even though the same exercise is often used across micro-cycles and meso-cycles.

Bass's "Ripped Cycle System"* is shown in Table 3.

TABLE 3

Phase	Time	Reps	Sets	Performance	Volume	Intensity
Endurance	4 weeks	15–25	1–2+	Slow, continuous	High	Low
Strength/ Endurance	4 weeks	10–15	1–2+	Moderate speed with pause	Moderate	Moderate
Strength	4 weeks	6–10	1–2+	Explosive	Low	High

+After warm-up sets   *Adapted from Bass, 1986, p. 97.

In Bass's approach, several different exercises may be done per body part, but for only one to two sets after a warm-up. This provides more variety, may provide a better training stimulus, and reduces boredom. It is also important to note that "explosive" repetitions do *not* mean flinging weights around. That is a sure way to injury. Rather, explosive means performing repetitions with some speed and a pause between repetitions, always having the weight under control.

Periodization and Aerobic Training

As I noted before and as Bass has detailed, this same scheme works well with aerobic training. For example, Table 4 shows two model track workouts, one each for the endurance and the strength phase.

The endurance workout features six repetitions of between three quarters and one quarter mile at about 80 percent capacity. The interval is kept at a quarter mile because the repetitions are only done at 80 percent capacity. With a warm-up and cool-down of a mile each, the total workout is about six and a half miles. The strength workout has five repetitions of between one half to one eighth of a mile (220 m), but at 90

TABLE 4

Phase	Warm-up	Rep Scheme	Pace	Interval	Cool Down	Total Distance
Endurance	1 mile	3/4, 1/2, 1/4, 1/4, 1/2, 3/4	About 80% of capacity at that distance	1/4 mile	1 mile	About 6.5 miles
Strength	1 mile	1/2, 1/4, 1/8 (220), 1/8 (220), 1/4	About 90–95% of capacity at that distance	1/2 mile	1 mile	About 5.5 miles

percent to 95 percent of capacity. The interval is kept relatively long (one half mile) so that maximum effort can be put into each repetition. With the one-mile warm-up and cool-down, the total workout is only about five and a half miles.

Obviously all the points made about gradual, ascending goals through a micro-cycle pertain here. For example, if the goal pace for a quarter mile during the endurance phase is 80 seconds, Week One's quarter mile repetitions would probably be run in 86 seconds. That is, the runner would reduce the time a few seconds per week. However, recalling the graph in the first part of this chapter, the start of a new phase calls for a bit of backing off. For example, let's say an athlete ended up a Strength/Endurance cycle at 75 seconds per quarter. The athlete is aiming for 72-second quarters in the strength phase. It is recommended that he or she start the strength phase by backing off to 77-second quarters.

Advantages of Periodization

Periodization allows the athlete to plan and do workouts that have very specific objectives, for example, to do a certain number of repetitions with a specific weight in a movement or to run a certain distance at a specific pace. Fulfilling the objectives means the workout is a success and is completed. Therefore, as will be discussed in a moment, overly long or frequent workouts are not called for—indeed, they are counterproductive.

It should also be obvious that the periodization system works well for athletes who enjoy being very meticulous and systematic in their training. Keeping detailed records and using those records to plan different workouts is one key aspect of making periodization continue to work. This may appear to take a lot of effort and to take some of the fun and spontaneity out of training. As we will see, continued progress *does* provide a lot of fun and satisfaction. And, in my own experience, "spontaneous" workouts were only occasionally satisfying, and worse, sometimes led to injury.

Before seeing why periodization works so well from a psychological perspective, let's take a lengthy excursion and examine recent work on training variables and routines that complement periodization.

AN EXCURSION INTO TRAINING

A number of, but certainly not all, masters athletes report increased difficulty with recovery from hard training in their 40s and 50s. It is unclear if decreased recovery ability is a natural result of aging, a result of less than optimal training, or perhaps both. Probably all readers of this book are aware that today virtually all athletes use a hard day-easy day training program. Progress is better when hard training days are followed by easy days, which may mean complete rest or lower level training. Such an approach is ideal for masters athletes, but many readers may be less sure about how hard to make hard days, how easy to make easy days, how frequently training should occur, and how long a training session should run.

Frequency and Intensity

For weight training, there is growing evidence that working body parts hard once per week and once easy leads to the best progress for most people. The "hard" session should be at goal weights and repetitions set up in your periodization program. The "easy" session should be at about 85 percent of the goal weight for that week, but with the same number of repetitions. If there is a problem with recovery, easy session weights may be reduced to 80 percent, or even 75 percent or 70 percent.

For the person using weight training as an adjunct to other activities, this means that they can do two whole body workouts a week, one at 100 percent and one at 85 percent or less. Alternate plans where weight training is the main activity, such as for bodybuilding, are shown in Table 5 (adapted from Bass, 1986).

TABLE 5

	Days			
Plan 1	1		3	5
	Whole Body Workout "A" 100%		Whole Body Workout "B" 80–90%	Whole Body Workout "A" 80%
Plan 2	1		3	5
	Upper Body Workout 100%		Lower Body Workout 100%	Total Body Workout 85%
Plan 3	1	2	3	5 (or 6)
	Chest and Upper Back 100%	Legs and Lower Back 100%	Shoulders and Arms 100%	Total Body Workout 85%

For these routines, the days refer to days within a week. Days not listed for workouts are off days.

Other variations of these routines can easily be developed (see Appendix B), and, in some cases, better results will occur when a training cycle (the hard and easy workouts) unfolds over an eight/nine day period. In addition, a number of people, including myself, have found that because deadlifts are so taxing, they should be done only once a week in the hard session. Aerobic and weight training sessions should also complement each other. For example, on a day you work your upper body with weights, you can use a rower for aerobics. On a lower-body day, you can cycle or run, and on a whole-body day, you can use a ski machine, an Air Dyne, or power walk with weights.

While both weight and aerobic training follow periodization, you should only really push extra hard on the one activity you want most to improve. Available evidence indicates you are unlikely to be outstanding in a strength and aerobic activity at the *same* time. You need to make a choice. Finally, off days for any routine should include just a relaxing activity such as easy walking.

What about the frequency of aerobic workouts for aerobic athletes? For a number of years, I have tried to make the case that there should be some real similarities in the training variables of strength and endurance athletes. Yet, in the 1970s while strength athletes were emphasizing relatively infrequent, short, intense sessions, aerobic athletes, particularly runners, were doing more and more volume. The "junk-mile era" seems to be over, and runners are starting to emphasize more quality, and even (to some, heretically) advocating *not* running every day.

Although I readily admit it is next to impossible to find a top runner who trains that way, I am quite confident that creative variations on Plan One in Table 5 would do the job for most top runners and endurance athletes. This would be especially true if the athlete followed a periodization approach, made the 100 percent session really taxing, focused on interval training geared to events they wanted to excel in, and actually took the off days. Some experts will tell you this approach was tried in the 1940s and 1950s and "it didn't work." What they often fail to note is that athletes of that era were often doing hard intervals five or six times per week and not following a periodization model. No wonder "it didn't work."

One athlete whose training of necessity approximated this approach was Roger Bannister, the first runner to break the four-minute barrier in the mile (see also Tracy Smith's training program, p. 220). Bannister was in medical school and didn't have much time to train, so he spent only about three hours per week on quality workouts.

Although by "modern standards," his workouts constituted a mere warm-up, his training may have been the most efficient of all time. Do you have any doubt that with better shoes and track surface and a psychological barrier at, say, 3:50, Bannister would have run the mile seven or eight seconds faster?

The periodization model and all the points made about training intensity and frequency also pertain to the health and fitness buff. If you enjoy a string of lower-level workouts and still see yourself improving, then stick with what you are doing. However, as Jan and Terry Todd have noted, boredom leads many fitness enthusiasts to lose that spark and drop out. So, for example, the jogger or walker, instead of doing those four or five workouts per week at the same moderate pace, should try doing three systematic workouts per week (see Table 5) that are different, interesting, and challenging.

It is easy to summarize everything said so far about training frequency and intensity. Do not train intensely very often, but when you do, make it a hard, systematic session that follows a periodization plan.

Duration

What about duration? How long should workouts be? Unless you are training for a marathon, there is no reason to do very long workouts. In fact, even if you are a marathoner, you probably only need to have one long workout every week or 10 days.

As the psychological perspective in Chapter 2 and the periodization approach indicate, workouts should be set up so you are successful and so the activity is most often enjoyable and almost always satisfying. A good prescription is to make your main training focus no more than an hour and any other activity about a half hour. For example, my four weight workouts each week average about one hour and my aerobic workouts take 30 minutes plus a 5-minute warm-up and cool-down.

Do not make the mistake of continually adding extra time and activity to your workouts. Since it is safe to say that many athletes overtrain, a good adage is when in doubt about your training and its effectiveness, do *less*, but try to do it more *intensely*.

A second adage comes from Clarence Bass: "Training

should be enjoyable, not something you dread." In Chapter 2, it was emphasized that, while of course environments and schedules influence people, many of us have it within our power to alter our environments. If your training is not interesting and challenging, *change it*. A good start is working out somewhat different goals in your periodization program so that your feedback is more positive and your success more meaningful.

Maintenance

According to Frank Zane (see pp 243–249), there is no such thing as "maintenance." You are either going in one direction or another.

In one sense, Frank is right. In training and in any activity in life, it is difficult to just stand still. Such a stance is not very interesting or challenging and, hence, it often does not work.

However, there are some good indications that fitness and strength can be maintained. You can pretty well maintain your speed in a two-mile run or your poundage in a bench press, if you do the right things. In addition, it appears possible to maintain one activity or movement while improving another.

An excellent series of studies by Dr. Robert C. Hickson, a professor in the College of Health, Physical Education, and Recreation at the University of Illinois at Chicago, sheds light on the critical variables in maintenance. In his studies, subjects were trained at high intensities for 10 weeks, on alternate days of fast, continuous running for 40 minutes and six, five-minute repetitions with two-minute rest intervals on stationary bikes. Heart rates during the six sessions per week were in the 90 percent plus range.

After this initial training period, subjects in different studies either reduced training frequency, duration, or intensity by one-third or two-thirds during an additional 15-week training period. That is, each subject was only involved in one training variable manipulation, for example, reducing duration by one-third.

Although there were many measures in these different studies, the most important results were presented graphically by Dr. Hickson as a composite of the three studies. The figure below shows an adaption of the results across the studies for the effects on treadmill VO_2 uptake, a measure of VO_2 max, after 10 weeks of training, and then after 15 weeks of reduced training. The bold line represents subjects training at a one-third reduction, and the thin line represents a two-thirds reduction. Although not shown, the results for maximum VO_2 uptake on a cycle were similar.

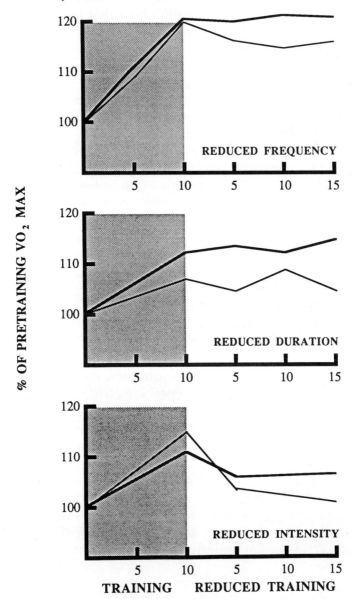

Overall, it is quite clear that a one-third reduction in frequency or duration had little effect, and, indeed, even a two-thirds reduction in these two variables had very minimal effects on the VO_2 max measure represented as a percent of pretraining levels. Reduced intensity had a larger impact on the VO_2 max. Indeed, Hickson and his colleagues concluded that: "When taken together and in relation to the training protocol employed, these results show that training intensity plays a principle role in regulating the maintenance of the increased aerobic power" (Hickson, R. C., et al. Reduced training intensities and loss of aerobic power, endurance, and cardiac growth. *Journal of Applied Physiology*, 58, 492–99).

Dr. Hickson pointed out that a training regime designed to acquire aerobic capacity probably differs from one designed for maintenance. For example, only running two days per week may not be enough to maximize aerobic fitness. However, once a capacity is acquired, it may be maintained by less frequent or long sessions, *if* some of those sessions are of high intensity.

Interestingly, these results parallel those reported in the introductory chapter from Dr. Pollock's longitudinal study. Recall that competitive men who maintained intensity (speed) in their running maintained measures of fitness across the 10-year test period and generally across their middle years. The noncompetitive men who maintained volume, but not intensity, showed a drop-off in fitness measures.

Although apparently there are no similar studies on strength and weight training, it is quite likely that maintenance of strength is also most related to intensity. For example, to be able to continue to squat 10 repetitions with 320 pounds, it is probable that once every week to 10 days a person would have to do at least one hard set of squats. It may be that at the end of an endurance phase in a periodization plan, the person would do one set at 280 pounds for 20 repetitions, and after a strength phase, one set at 345 pounds for 6 repetitions. That will probably maintain the ability to do 320 pounds for 10 repetitions. However, it is almost certain that doing four, five, or six sets of 10 repetitions with 220 pounds will *not* maintain the ability to do 320 pounds for 10 repetitions.

Thus, in many ways, we have come full circle. The best way to improve or maintain is to train briefly, relatively infrequently, but quite intensely. And, the best way to array these training variables and to accomplish training goals is through following a periodization program. Now let's turn to understanding why periodization works so well from a psychological perspective.

PSYCHOLOGICAL UNDERPINNING OF PERIODIZATION

A number of the psychological terms used in Chapter 2 are briefly reintroduced here. Recall that *self-efficacy* referred to a person's belief in the ability to perform specific actions under particular conditions. *Outcome expectancy* is essentially a person's belief that following certain plans will lead to designated desirable outcomes, that following the program will result in predictable benefits. These two beliefs are central to motivation.

Feedback and *goal setting* were procedures based on formal or informal processes that also were essential for maintaining a high level of motivation and performance. Feedback on performance in relationship to specific goals can be generated by external sources, such as a coach or training partner. More often, and particularly for masters athletes, feedback is self-generated for goals picked by the athlete. Particular goals are closely related to personal standards, and feedback is tied into self-evaluative, cognitive, and affective processes. Feedback tells us how well we have surpassed, met, or failed to reach our personal standards.

It can be quickly seen that an ideal training system would be set up in such a way that:

1. Self-efficacy beliefs are maintained at a high level.
2. Outcome expectancy is high because progress is visible— the system works.
3. Goals are hard, but reachable, and over time become higher.
4. Feedback is almost always positive.

Periodization fits all of these points. However, before expanding on them it is instructive to observe what happens when a system does not take these points into account.

Training to "Failure"

For many years, I followed the advice of Arthur Jones (the founder of Nautilus), and for most of my weight training sessions I trained to "failure." What that means is that every exercise was carried to the point where another repetition was not possible. You literally failed. Obviously, from a psychological perspective, the term "fail" is not a wise one to use. Jones could have said, "When you can no longer do another repetition, you have 'succeeded.' " I do not feel this is just playing with words. Words guide our feelings, thoughts, and self-evaluations, so it *does* make a good deal of difference what words are used—whether I could say that I failed or succeeded.

But the major difficulty is what I call the "encore problem." What do you do in the next workout? I recall doing a number of workouts and, following Jones's advice, collapsing at their conclusion. In fact, I particularly recall a workout that concluded with high-repetition, stiff-leg deadlifts. I collapsed in place after that last set and it took about 20 minutes to revive myself. How do you top that effort? And, indeed, there's a worse part of training to utter failure. Usually, you approach the next workout with a feeling that is best described as *dread*. How do you motivate yourself over the long haul to do something again and again that is unbelievably hard and painful? The answer is that no one really knows.

Common sense and psychology tell us that motivating yourself to do hard, challenging, but enjoyable workouts is a relatively easy task. With periodization you greatly look forward to the next workout instead of dreading it. In a real sense, periodization redefines what is meant by intensity. Intensity is found in the slow buildup and gradually ascending goals, not in a few unreal, gut-busting workouts.

Choosing Training Goals

Thus, periodization, if it is to be optimized, really revolves around correctly picking training goals. This usually takes one meso-cycle because you can familiarize yourself with your ability at different intensity and volume ranges. In the following micro-cycles and meso-cycles, your goals should be correct and you should be improving upon your performances in the next meso-cycle.

What is a correct goal? A correct goal is a performance that, with a several week buildup and a concerted, focused effort, you can reach with about a 90 percent probability in the last workout of a micro-cycle. It is an effort that you can feel good about and represents sustained, although often modest, improvement. To put this in perspective, I feel that if I can add two and a half pounds in an upper body movement and five pounds for a lower body movement each meso-cycle, then I have picked a suitable goal and am showing improvement. For a seasoned runner, improving as little as one second per quarter-mile repetition would represent a good goal.

These sound like very small increments, and they are. The overall objective in periodization is to be able to make such improvements over a very long period of time. For example, after six meso-cycles, an athlete who bench pressed 205 and squatted 350, both for six repetitions, would now be able to bench press 220 six times and squat for 380 six times. Likewise, a runner starting with 90-second quarters, a 6-minute pace, might get down to 82-second quarters, better than a 5:30 pace.

At this point, it should be clear exactly how to set up and develop a periodization approach for various training activities. It should also start to become clear how the system fits with psychological principles of motivation. Table 6 (p. 74) summarizes how key psychological principles mesh with the periodization system.

What Periodization Will and Won't Do

It is important at this juncture to mention some qualifying points. Periodization is not magical. It will not change a person with ordinary genetic potential into a superstar. It is a system, however, that will take you closer to that elusive "fulfillment of your potential."

TABLE 6

Psychological Principle	Periodization System
Self-effficacy	With gradually ascending goals, athletes know with a high degree of certainty that all workouts will be successfully completed.
Outcome expectancy	Progress in the short and long run is almost always visible. Confidence in the program is maintained.
Goals	Goals are intelligently developed based on experience. Goals are hard, but reachable and ascending.
Feedback	Feedback, success in meeting goals, is almost always positive. Positive feedback means workouts are challenging and enjoyable, a positive affect is maintained, and personal standards are fulfilled.

Periodization is also not a system that will work well without environmental supports. As was noted in Chapter 2, training cannot be optimized without proper scheduling of workouts and recuperation, relaxation, and reasonably good nutrition. In other words, introducing periodization haphazardly will not work. Indeed, it should be apparent that periodization is a highly planned system that virtually demands a well-ordered life to fully function.

However, there is "another hand" to this assessment. Rarely does a training system so closely match psychological principles. And it is even rarer that maximizing all aspects of the training system maximizes all key psychological principles. Thus, it appears that with periodization the possibilities exist for highly synergistic effects. Physical and psychological variables interact in unique and optimal ways so that you can reach new heights of performance and achievement.

Now that you know how to optimize the physical/behavioral aspects of training, it is time to use the same principles to optimize cognitions and affect necessary for top training and competition.

4

Focused Concentration: The Real Way to Learn This Valuable Skill

INTRODUCTION TO MENTAL TRAINING

No one who engages in training and sports can dispute that our thoughts and feelings greatly influence performance by setting or removing constraints to optimal behavior. Two of my own experiences are interesting illustrations of the general phenomenon, and, doubtless, readers can provide a number of their own examples.

The first example is a dramatic one, but it has happened a number of times to me. This particular instance occurred about 20 years ago. My last exercise in a workout was stiff-leg deadlifts. I was supposed to try to do 15 repetitions with 300 pounds. Because I was tired and lethargic, I decided that instead I would do 5 or 6 reps with 325 pounds, which in some ways is an easier effort. I loaded the bar and, without much focus and enthusiasm, lifted the weight. It felt pretty heavy, but I continued and finished the 5 reps, thankful that the workout was done.

The last thing I had to do before hitting the shower was to unload the bar and generally straighten out my home gym. When I stacked up the weights, the stacks looked big. I found I had actually lifted 375 pounds five times, a feat I had not accomplished before or, unfortunately, since that point.

The second example is more commonplace. It happened about a year ago. Part of our basement was being redone and carpeted. I had wanted to finish my aerobic workout in the gym side of the basement before all the commotion started, but that wasn't possible. Also, much to my dismay, all the furniture in the finished part had been placed in the gym area. The windows and door were open, it was cold, and workmen were bringing things in and out of the basement and hammering away. Instead of becoming angry and emotional, I told myself, "Stay calm. There's nothing you can do. Just do the best you can."

My ski machine, the aerobic exercise for the day, was surrounded by furniture and boxes. It felt like I was enclosed in a telephone booth when I got on the machine. I started my routine and just concentrated on staying relaxed and doing my workout plan. I was able to block out most of my surroundings. Forty minutes later, I was done. It was a great workout! As I got off the machine to find a place to stretch, I again noticed all the clutter, noise, and commotion.

The first example shows how the mind (i.e., our beliefs) often sets limits that are much below our real physical potential. If in some way the mind can be harnessed, or even fooled, we are probably capable of performances far beyond our day-to-day activity. The second example is much more commonplace, but shows how more positive thoughts, a relaxed state, and focused concentration can enhance performance even under much less than ideal circumstances.

Most of this chapter pertains to this second kind of experience. However, much of what will be said also has relevance for surpassing limits set by our own beliefs, as in the first example.

Readers also know and have experienced the other side of the coin. Doubt, negative self-statements, and anxiety can lead the most able athlete to lousy workouts and abysmal competitions. Thus, the case for enlisting cognitive and affective processes into athletic training and competition is a strong one. However, both as a research psychologist and an athlete, I feel it is important to move away from the almost cultish manner in which so-called "mental training" has been presented to coaches, athletes, and the public.

The purpose of this chapter is three-fold. The processes involved in mental training need to be demystified. An orderly framework for understanding those processes will be developed. And, an individualized approach to such training based on the framework and other points from Chapter 2 needs to be articulated.

DEMYSTIFYING MENTAL TRAINING

This section begins with a series of "not" statements. This is necessary because mental training *has* often been presented in a simplified, yet hyped, way as a psychological panacea.

- Mental training is not necessarily the incarnation of the power of Eastern ways, much less occult or mysterious forces.
- Mental training will not lead to miracles. An average athlete will not reach startling heights of achievement, and almost certainly will not become a champion.
- The skills involved in acutely using cognitive and affective processes should not be enlisted for all training sessions.
- As with any other cognitive and affective processes and behavior, these abilities do not occur in a vacuum.
- There is a specific theory, literature, and research that relates to mental training. It is not an isolated set of procedures and techniques.
- Mental training is not sports psychology in its entirety, although some practitioners and the public unfortunately believe this to be the case.

It is now appropriate to be more positive and say what mental training is and what it can do.

- Mental training uses some established principles and techniques from social-cognitive theory and behavioral psychology.

- Mental training can help the average and excellent athlete enhance performance when it is used as an adjunct to physical training.
- Optimal use of cognitive and affective skills is affected by other aspects of our lives and by our environment.
- Active engagement of high-level cognitive and affective skills should be reserved for especially hard workouts and competitions, although learning and practice of these skills must take place under realistic circumstances.
- The same framework developed in Chapter 2 to study, describe, and prescribe motivational processes and techniques is appropriate for defining and detailing mental training strategies.

FRAMEWORK FOR MENTAL TRAINING

The term *mental training* means a set of techniques to focus attention, lower anxiety, and provide one or more procedures to refocus or divert attention. In Chapter 2, these skills were referred to as *focused concentration*.

Thus, we are describing interrelated behaviors that are connected to the cognitive, affective, and environmental domains. If your first response to the prior point is, "But isn't that exactly how we started to look at athletic motivation in Chapter 2?" you are right. It does not make sense to switch theory and framework to fit every nuance of behavior. And, a good theory and framework is adaptable for many different kinds of phenomena.

In Figure 1 we see the interactive systems model that was described in detail in Chapter 2. Let us now look at each element and see what is necessary to reach the goals of focused attention, decreased anxiety, and refocusing attention.

Many athletes report that optimal performance occurs when they are in a state that is characterized by both calmness and heightened vigilance. Interestingly, these frequent reports are different from the idea of being terrifically "psyched

FIGURE 1

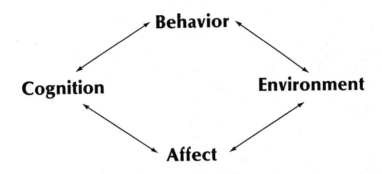

up." An image that comes to mind is football players pounding each other or running into locker walls prior to a game. Even though the sport is violent, it doesn't appear that equally violent psyching up is appropriate, and it is probably very inappropriate for most other sports.

There is a classic performance-arousal curve that substantiates this position. Up to a point, arousal and anxiety facilitate performance. As arousal and anxiety increase, performance, particularly on complex tasks, rapidly decreases. Thus, the power lifter or sprinter may be helped to a point by a reasonable level of arousal. That same level of arousal, however, may be detrimental to a gymnast, golfer, tennis player, or quarterback. Thus, for most sports, only a moderate, controlled level of arousal and anxiety is appropriate.

My own experience follows the classic arousal-performance curve. Almost all the PRs (personal record) that I have ever made in weight training occurred when I felt focused, but relaxed. In fact, the PRs almost always felt easy. Conversely, when I got "psyched up," I almost always failed to achieve the PR. Thus, many athletes need to learn how to relax and stay calm under tough training and competition conditions. Fortunately, learning relaxation responses, at least initially, is not that difficult. Several techniques work, and one of these, cue controlled relaxation, is described in Appendix A.

All the techniques start with fairly long and elaborate procedures. With practice—and as shown in Appendix A, it *does* take a good deal of practice—many athletes can learn to put themselves in a relaxed state in a matter of moments. As we will see in the last sections of this chapter, learning the initial relaxation response is a critical step, but not the only one. The various steps involved in the "transfer of training" (applying skills learned in a special situation to other situations) are also extremely important.

Not everyone can learn to relax equally well. People differ in what is called *trait anxiety*, their reactions to particular situations (*state anxiety*), and their ability to master relaxation skills. However, when athletes do learn a relaxation response, it can have some very good reciprocal and what we called in Chapter 2 "reverberating" effects. We can now turn to the cognitive domain to look at some of those effects.

Cognitive Domain

What is particularly important is that athletes believe that they have an effective method to control anxiety (remember how we defined *outcome expectancy*) and that they are capable of using the control strategy in the specific circumstances where and when it is needed (recall the term *self-efficacy*). These beliefs become sharpened when initial training in relaxation is successful and when the first attempts to use the strategy "for real" are also successful. Proper staging of practice is a key procedure that will be discussed later.

Cognitive processes also entail other self-regulatory mechanisms. For example, through practice athletes can learn to self-monitor their mood and make some judgements about it that then lead to specific changes. A tennis player should be able to monitor not only form, but also how anxious she is feeling. A properly trained tennis player can lower anxiety during a match to achieve more optimal performance.

The entire process is the same as the ones in the second chapter where we described personal standards, self-observations, self-judgements, and self-reactions. Additional cognitive strategies involved in learning and practicing relaxation will include visualization techniques, which are also described later.

Behavioral Domain

Two sets of behaviors are most important in focusing attention. The first set includes those behaviors related to relaxation. These are the actual relaxation responses and any cues (e.g., self-statements such as the word *calm*) or other devices (e.g., focused, deep breathing) used to initiate or alter the relaxation response. The second set of behaviors is sometimes forgotten by athletes and coaches. What exactly are the athletic behaviors that are called for, and how will the relaxation responses fit with these behaviors?

Athletic behaviors differ on such dimensions as skill requirements (i.e., complexity as in the arousal-performance curve), duration, degree of effort, and bandwidth of attention (see Chapter 2). For example, gymnastics requires a very high degree of skill, displayed for short periods of time (30 seconds to 2 minutes), but with maximum effort and usually a very narrow focus of attention. Marathon running does not require great skill but does call for a moderate to high effort over hours, also with a narrow focus. Power lifting involves low skill, explosive effort for seconds, with a narrow focus. Quarterbacking requires high skill, intermittent moderate to high effort over an extended time, and narrow and wide foci of attention. The important behavioral parameters of sports and examples are shown in Table 1 (p. 82).

Thus, the requirements of any sport have to be analyzed and the exact training and practice of relaxation and focused concentration fitted to the sport. Of course, when the fit is a good one and the procedures actually work, affect (mood and emotion) will be modulated, self-regulatory practices will be given a proper field of play, outcome expectancy and self-efficacy

TABLE 1
IMPORTANT BEHAVIORAL DIMENSIONS OF CONTRASTING SPORTS

Sport	Skill Requirement	Duration	Effort	Attention Bandwidth
Gymnastics	High; Intricate	Routines last 30 to 90 seconds except for vaulting, but meets last for hours	Moderate to hard to explosive	Narrow
Marathon Running	Low	About 2 to 4 hours of continuous effort	Mostly high moderate to hard	Very narrow except for tracking competition
Doubles Tennis	High	About 1 to 2 hours of intermittent effort	Intermittent moderate to hard; depends on game played	Narrow and moderately wide
Power Lifting	Low	Very short bursts of effort, meets last for hours	Explosive	Very narrow
Golf	High	Much time, but only limited time for actual play	Relaxed, power generation for drives and relaxed smooth play for putts	Narrow and moderately wide

beliefs will be enhanced and, overall, the ability to relax and focus concentration will be increased.

Environmental Domain

In the environmental domain, we analyze and explain more fully the tasks required in athletic behaviors, the settings in which the behaviors occur, and the obstacles to optimal performance. For the runner, a hilly course usually entails different adjustments than a straight or rolling course, and another set of adjustments is called for when running in extremes of weather. The golfer needs to analyze a host of environmental factors—terrain, slope, wind, distance—that differ for each hole. The game of tennis too, as demonstrated at Wimbledon each year, can vary depending upon the playing surface (e.g., grass versus clay or asphalt). These environmental variables alter what the athlete must do, and adjustments must be made to ensure the best performance under different circumstances.

Other important environmental factors include the nature of the game, e.g., if the athlete performs alone or with a partner or team, audience characteristics varying from a few spectators to packed arenas and international TV audiences, and the degree of competition. For example, in some sports, athletes largely compete against themselves although in comparison to others (e.g., bodybuilding and gymnastics). In other sports, athletes compete (and can interact) against one other person (e.g., singles tennis) or a few people (e.g., golf, weight lifting) or many people (e.g., road running). Competition also varies in intensity, i.e., the importance of a match, meet, or race, the qualities and abilities of opponents, and the degree of actual interaction with opponents.

Other environmental variables are more easily described as psychosocial characteristics of the setting as perceived by the athlete. In an interesting article about anxiety and sports performance, Bradley Hatfield and Gerald Walford (Understanding anxiety: implications for sports performance *National Strength and Conditioning Association Journal*, April/May,

1987, 9(2), 58–65) described some critical perceptions. These were:

- The perceived importance of the competition, which can be quite different for individuals and team members.
- The perceived discrepancy between the athlete's abilities and the standard of success. The discrepancy between skills and standards may be accurately or inaccurately perceived in positive directions (skills are overestimated) or negative directions (skills are underestimated).
- The perceived negative consequences of failure, which also may be accurate or inaccurate.

Each environmental condition and perception of the environment will often engender different responses and different needs as far as maintaining a state of focused concentration. For example, the gymnast competing at a small, quickly run, national-level competition on national TV, who underestimates her skills and dreads failure, will probably require somewhat different strategies than when she is competing in a slowly paced local competition seen only by a few people, where she knows her skills are tops and where she will undoubtedly win.

These points indicate that practice of focused concentration must be made *specific* to behavioral and environmental circumstances, a point to be addressed in the next sections of this chapter. However, one other point will be made here. Often, athletes will be pushed, by themselves and by their coaches, to use extraordinary focused-concentration skills and other strategies as an ingredient of their daily training. In part, this is done by always making the training very hard. But as we discussed at length in the chapter on periodization, such a method of training is almost always counterproductive from both psychological and physiological perspectives.

The need for using extraordinary focused concentration skills can be controlled by modulating the training regime. Intuitively, a good time to practice focused concentration skills is at the end of each micro-training cycle when large efforts are required and/or simulated competitions are conducted.

INDIVIDUALIZED TRAINING

This section provides the principles and procedures of a step-by-step approach to training in focused concentration and related abilities. The approach is based on the framework used throughout this book plus some additional points.

Assessment

By now it should be clear that any mental training program needs to be individualized in at least two ways. First, the specific cognitive, affective, behavioral, and environmental aspects of the sport have to be understood. This means that although in *principle* the "mental training" programs of diverse athletes such as gymnasts, golfers, tennis players, and runners are the same, the actual training program and particular use of the strategies will differ. Second, the specific problems of the athlete need to be assessed. For example, one golfer may have difficulty sustaining attention during a long round of golf when he perceives dire consequences for a high score, while another golfer becomes very anxious when playing difficult holes or when the score is close and she perceives that her competition's skills are superior to hers.

From this perspective, there is not a prepackaged "mental training program for golfers or runners," but rather a set of principles for devising an individualized program. Thus, after the specific requisites of the sport are understood, further individualized assessment is necessary.

Individual assessment follows the framework. It provides the specific information pertinent to environmental circumstances, behaviors, feelings, thoughts, and perceptions. You can gather this information primarily through structured interviews with the athlete. Additional information can be obtained from the athlete's coach, but, of course, such an interview should be secured by permission of the athlete. Much of the information can and should come from self-monitoring. In fact, by following the guidelines of this chapter many athletes can do their own assessments.

First, the athlete needs to know what, *exactly*, are the circumstances where the problems of anxiety, inattention, doubt, or feelings of loss of control manifest themselves. The answer is not, "When I'm in a tough singles match," but rather, "When I'm in a singles match with a player with a strong serve and volley game, when the score is tied or I am behind, and when there are people watching."

Second, under these circumstances, what exactly are you thinking, feeling, and doing? Again, this information must be very specific. For example, the tennis player under the circumstances described above may start telling himself he is going to lose the match, and worse, make a fool of himself; start feeling very anxious, which for this person means that his mind starts racing and he feels tension all over his body but particularly in his legs and arms; and begin playing a conservative, defensive, baseline game which is not his game at all. As his game deteriorates and he falls further behind, negative thoughts and feelings, such as acute doubts about his skills, become worse, following the downward spiralling schema discussed in Chapter 2.

In sports where there are breaks, an athlete can keep a self-monitoring log of circumstances, thoughts, feelings, and behaviors. An example of such a log is shown in Table 2. In sports where this is not possible, a self-monitoring log should be completed immediately after the practice, event, or competition.

Note how specific and detailed the log is. The athlete has even been asked to rate his concentration and anxiety levels in situations, a practice that is useful for both assessment and intervention. In addition, note that anxiety-provoking situations may occur well before the actual meet or match. These "antecedent" situations, thoughts, feelings, and behaviors must also be emphasized in anxiety reduction and focused-concentration training. Therefore, a self-monitoring log, such

TABLE 2

SELF-MONITORING LOG OF A COMPETITIVE MASTERS TENNIS PLAYER

Situation (#)	What thinking?	Concentration Level (1–10)	How feeling?	Anxiety Level (1–10)	What doing?	Self-control/ coping
4. At home, in bed trying to sleep; about 11 p.m.	About the upcoming (3 days away) match; whether I'll choke or not	4; my mind is racing about all parts of the match	Some anxiety and dread	6	Tossing & turning; got up and read for 15 minutes	The reading, also trying to think about other things (not successful)
10. After the match; Tied at 1 set each in best of 3 match; score was 2–3 in games with opponent serving	My game is going to collapse; I'm going to choke again. I'll start making a lot of errors; people will laugh at me.	2; can't concentrate on just playing; I'm concentrating on losing	Starting to get very anxious	8½	Starting to play defensively, baseline game	Telling myself be calm but aggressive; not working

as that in Table 2, should be kept for two to four weeks, enough time to experience and record critical situations.

Interviews with athletes can be an adjunct to the self-monitoring log by helping to "flesh out" the log and to review other relevant material not in the log or experienced after the log is completed. In addition, two other assessment techniques are very useful. An athlete, alone or with help, can actively visualize difficult situations and describe the setting and his various responses in detail. Even better, the athlete can role play the difficult situations and note specific reactions. For example, you can get on the tennis court and role play the situation described previously. Such techniques will also be useful in early training phases described a bit later.

More than likely, there will be gradations of situations and responses. For example, when the tennis player's opponent has a less powerful game and the score has seesawed, negative responses may be minimal. However, for some athletes it is actually anticipation that elicits the most anxiety, negative feelings, and inappropriate behaviors (see Table 2). For example, the golfer may start to ruminate about a match days before the event, and the closer the event gets, the worse the anxiety. Such high anticipatory anxiety leads to an array of maladaptive responses and subpar performance. Likewise, the athlete's perceptions of particular situations, and how close they come to reality, need to be assessed. This type of assessment is usually best done with a second, objective party.

In any case, at the end of the assessment stage, which can require several hours of effort in conversation, role playing, visualization, and self-monitoring in real-life settings, the athlete should have an excellent handle on both the specific requirements of the sport and the individual's specific reactions to specific circumstances. The training phases can now begin.

Training Phases

Training must fit the particular circumstances and problems of the athlete. However, in addition, as briefly explained in Chapter 2, training also needs to follow a relatively orderly sequence of phases. The phases are *acquisition, generality,* and *sustained.*

The acquisition phase is often the only phase of many training programs. Here, usually with considerable time and effort, the athlete learns the skills that are needed. Often, this training may be done under artificial conditions. For example, much of the training may occur in an office setting through visualization trials. There may only be a few real-life trials with the new skills.

In some cases, only these initial efforts may be required. However, when training does not also include the generality and sustained phases, there is frequently difficulty in maintaining the effective use of new skills. Often, the athlete is back where she started after a few weeks.

When all the phases are properly orchestrated, the likelihood of long-term success is much greater. There is also much more room for trial and error and fine-tuning procedures.

Figure 2 (pp. 90–91) shows a *process-of-change* schema for the different training phases and procedures for each phase. The schema is appropriate for any behavior change process, but here is applied to anxiety reduction and focused-concentration skills. The schema shows an unfolding process moving from intensive training using a range of techniques in a few situations to less intensive training with an emphasis on use and practice of skills under a variety of circumstances.

Another way of looking at the schema is that at first the emphasis is on learning the response and believing in the ability to use the new behaviors (self-efficacy) and their positive impacts (outcome expectancy). The later emphasis in training is use of new behaviors under different circumstances and incorporation of the beliefs into the athlete's self-standards, beliefs, and values. Of course, along the way, practice based on good examples (models) of the behaviors and with specific goals and feedback is very helpful. Each phase probably will be repeated in a step-by-step successive approximation to the goal of efficient and effective use of new behaviors.

In the acquisition phase, incentives may be used to start an anxious or reluctant athlete on the training process, with varying effectiveness. Modeling and role playing are extensively used to teach and practice skills resulting in high outcome

FIGURE 2

A PROCESS OF CHANGE SCHEMA

STAGES

Acquisition	Generality	Sustained
Processes & Procedures	Processes & Procedures	Processes & Procedures
Incentive (saliency, value, schedule, contingency) →	Modeling →	Self-efficacy →
Modeling (type, characteristics, number, outcomes) →	Self-efficacy →	Beliefs →
Role Play/Visualization →	Goal setting →	Values →
Outcome expectancies →	Staged practice in different settings →	Commitment (public, private) →
Self-efficacy →	Feedback →	Personal standards and self-regulatory processes
Goal Setting →	Modeling →	• Goals
Performance →	Self-efficacy →	• Self-feedback
	Goal setting →	• Self-evaluation
		• Self-reinforcement
		• Self-correction →

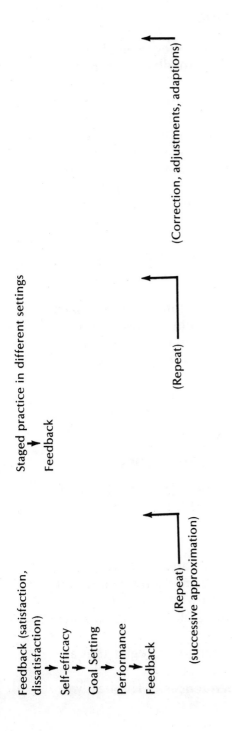

Feedback (satisfaction, dissatisfaction)
↓
Self-efficacy → Goal Setting → Performance → Feedback

(Repeat)
(successive approximation)

Staged practice in different settings
↓
Feedback

(Repeat)

(Correction, adjustments, adaptions)

expectancy, self-efficacy, and actual skill. Specific goals are set for practice sessions with, of course, feedback on performance an important ingredient. The process is repeated a number of times.

In the generality phase, similar procedures are used, but much more emphasis is placed on a step-by-step ("staged") approach to practice in increasingly difficult situations. Finally, in the sustained stage, the new skills are highly practiced, belief in the ability to use them is high, and their use and integration into sports training and competition and personal standards and self-regulatory processes are also very high. For example, an athlete may now perceive herself as able to stay calm and focused under *any* circumstance. That perception is now part of her values, and commitments to herself and others may be made based on this ability.

It also should be understood that a person may move back and forth through phases or be in different phases for different skills. For example, a person may find that her skills are not proficient enough to be used in many different situations. She may have to return to the acquisition phase. Or, an athlete may find that he can now maintain good concentration in any kind of practice session but must work further on acquiring skills to reduce anxiety in competitions.

DETAILED DESCRIPTION OF TRAINING

It is useful to describe some of the procedures and the rationale of each phase in a little more detail (see Figure 2).

Acquisition

The purpose of this phase is to efficiently and effectively learn new skills, or learn how to use skills gained under different circumstances. This phase starts after the assessment described above, when it is clear exactly what the athlete's problems and skill needs are.

We can outline several behavior change strategies that are emphasized in this phase.

Modeling/Role Playing/Feedback Sequences   The best way

to learn a skill is to first have that skill demonstrated by a competent individual. Second, the person learning the skill will try it out a number of times in a role play situation. On each trial, the person receives corrective feedback and perfects the skill. This sequence, when you think about it, is similar to the way most people learned how to drive.

Indeed, if you closely follow the entire process-of-change schema, it will resemble the steps and procedures in a good parent-led or school-based driver education program. For example, I recall how my dad showed me how to start, shift, and stop a car—over and over again. Next, my first venture behind the wheel occurred on a Sunday morning in an empty shopping mall parking lot. Sitting next to me, my dad provided encouragement and feedback. Over time, we drove together on neighborhood streets. Of course, later there were short solo trips, and so on, until the great day I drove alone into New York City, an accomplishment at any age!

There are variations to the acquisition sequence that are used when a person is essentially working alone and for skills that are internal—cognitive and affective control. In both instances, skills such as relaxation or the use of cue words (e.g., "focus") to instigate altered states of attention, must be practiced until the athlete can almost automatically relax and concentrate in nonthreatening situations such as the home. It is also important that practice sessions focus on important parts of the athlete's body, such as the hands for a golfer. Cue words ("calm," "focus") should also be paired with relaxation training (see Appendix B). In this way, the cue word will eventually elicit the relaxed and focused state.

The modeling part of this learning process comes into play when the athlete, for example, reads about the relaxation techniques and how other athletes have successfully used them. The athlete working alone may be able to enlist friends and other athletes for role playing sequences. On the other hand, because the techniques are internal, it is up to the athlete to self-observe internal thoughts (e.g., negative self-statements) and feelings (e.g., anxiety). On the other hand, there should always be some overt behavior that can also be used as an external indicator of how well the athlete is doing. For example, if the golfer is relaxed and concentrating, it would be expected that she would sink a good percentage of 10-foot putts.

When role playing is not possible, visualization strategies can be helpful. Different people have different degrees of skill in visualization, and for this strategy to work, a reasonable degree of skill is necessary. What you must be able to do is to actually visualize all important aspects of the situation and see yourself performing in them. If you can do that with enough involvement so that your thoughts and feelings are similar to the real situation, then visualization will be a helpful strategy for you.

Successive Approximation   As the term applies, this strategy entails a step-by-step sequence. In order to do this appropriately, the athlete in the assessment phase needs to be able to indicate a series of escalating troublesome circumstances. In practice, these may only be variations on the same theme. For example, for a diver it may be that with the increased intricacy of each dive and the increased importance of the meet come more negative thoughts and anxiety.

Once the athlete has a list of such specific situations—the list may be as short as 3 situations and as many as 20, including situations such as thinking about an upcoming race or match—they need to be ranked. What situations cause from the least to the most anxiety, negative thoughts, and inattention? Of course, these ratings should be based on the self-monitoring rating data (see Table 1).

As you might have guessed, the next step involves role playing and/or visualization, starting with the least troublesome situation and proceeding up a hierarchy of situations such as depicted in Table 3. The athlete should be using her cue words and relaxation responses for role play and/or visualization sessions. The athlete is only ready to move up to the next situation after thoughts, feelings, and behaviors have reached adequate levels. If, for example, an athlete is still anxious when visualizing a lower-level situation, it can mean two things: cue words and relaxation must be practiced more, or the situation is more threatening than realized (or both).

TABLE 3
HIERARCHY OF ANXIETY-PROVOKING SITUATIONS
FOR A COMPETITIVE MASTERS TENNIS PLAYER

Situation (#1)	Anxiety Level (1–10)
1. Signing up for the tournament two weeks from now at the City Tennis Pavilion	2
4. At home in bed trying to sleep, but thinking about upcoming match and choking	6
10. Tied at one set each in best of three match; score was 2–3 in games with opponent serving; thinking about choking; playing defensively	8½
14. Now down 2–4 in third set; just double-faulted to start game; thinking "I'm a 'choke artist' "	9½

Successive approximation is a strategy that nicely fits with many of the points and other strategies noted in Chapter 1. It usually leads to high self-efficacy because the athlete has a good sense that she can use the strategies effectively in the situation. Because self-efficacy is high, performance is usually good. Because performance is good, self-feedback and feedback from others is almost always positive. The process then increases self-efficacy about the ability to tackle the next situation and also increases outcome expectancies about the entire approach. If you see parallels and the same processes at work here as when we talked about the periodization approach to training (Chapter 3) and this chapter's example of learning to drive, you are exactly right.

Feedback/Goal Setting/Support   Feedback, goal setting, and social support are also important ingredients of a change program. As described in Chapter 2, the best system is setting up a series of hard but reachable goals and a simple feedback system that can show the athlete how close he came to reaching or surpassing those goals. In this instance, the goals can focus very much on the process and somewhat less on the outcomes. For example, goals can include keeping anxiety below a certain subjective level while visualizing a difficult part of a meet, or having only three negative self-statements during a role play of a tennis set, or being able to refocus attention within several seconds while visualizing running a long race. Goals can keep increasing in a number of ways. A goal can be to lower anxiety in increasingly more difficult (visualized) situations. A simple record system with specific goals, quite similar to a training dairy, can provide one form of feedback. Feedback can also come from friends, coaches, or other athletes who may be helping with the change process.

Additional elements involved in the change process are cognitive restructuring (being able to have a different perception of behaviors and circumstances) and social support. Feedback from an objective second party about the reality behind perceptions (e.g., regarding the skill level of the athlete and her competition) may be important where perceptions are off base and/or cause anxiety. For example, knowing that her skills are only passable but that she can win with her consistency may help an athlete who has accurately assessed her skills, but has unwarranted anxiety because of the assessment.

Social support can take many forms, but in essence it is having someone aware of what it is you are trying to do and being there to provide some empathy and encouragement. The person need not be an expert, another athlete, or coach, but simply someone who cares and whose caring you value.

Generality

This stage of training may be conducted during the last part of the acquisition stage or as a separate following stage. Basically, the same types of procedures and strategies are involved, but the emphasis is on using the techniques under different real-life circumstances. The athlete needs to use successive approximation in the generality phase in much the same way as he went through the hierarchy of situations in visualization and role play. Once a situation is mastered in the role play or visualization, it can be tried in real life.

Again, the generality phase makes use of modeling, feedback, goal setting, and support along with successive approximation, but the emphasis is a little bit different. The overall goal of the stage is to make the athlete able to effectively deal with a range of predictable and not-so-predictable situations. For example, the tennis player must be able to remain calm and focused against her opponent's strong serve and volley game even when the crowd favors the other player and her own first serve is off. Success in each more difficult situation means that a new situation can be tackled. If the athlete doesn't succeed, it may signify that the situation was too difficult or that for particular skills and situations the athlete must detour back to the acquisition stage.

Unfortunately, a good deal of cognitive and affective training ends at the acquisition stage. The athlete will practice a fair amount with visualization and then be sent forth into competition. It's as if my dad sent me to drive on the interstate directly after my tour of the parking lot! Obviously, in almost all cases this is a mistake and will result in failure and setbacks. The generality stage needs to be planned with as much thought as the acquisition stage and the athlete's overall training program.

Sustained

As this term implies, the athlete uses the effective cognitive and affective strategies not only in various situations but over a long period of time. The ability to use such strategies and the performance that results are now firmly part of the athlete's personal standards and self-regulatory processes. For example, a personal standard of the golfer may be that regardless of the course, competition, or weather, she will always remain calm and focused. Or the runner's personal standard includes being able to run long distances just below an anaerobic threshold while maintaining a relaxed but vigilant state. The skills are part of the athlete's value system.

Most importantly, these new personal standards and values will be based on firm outcome and efficacy beliefs and, of course, performance. Past experience substantiates the beliefs and standard. In turn, the athlete will formally or informally monitor the strategies and react to them in a manner described in detail in Chapter 2.

This may mean that over time there will be a need for fine-tuning or even a complete refresher course as new situations and performance demands arise. The adaptation and learning process should really never end. Hopefully, by following the framework, principles, and procedures of this chapter, athletes will find adaptation and learning more systematic, effective, and enjoyable.

5
Portraits of Ageless Athletes

INTRODUCTION TO THE PORTRAITS

The most exciting part of doing this book was the opportunity to talk and correspond in depth with exemplar masters athletes. I had followed the careers of some of these individuals for many years, while some of the others I only became acquainted with by doing this book. As I mentioned in the first chapter, I was also fortunate in that five of these athletes lived almost in my own backyard.

The 17 athletes portrayed in this book nicely represent masters athletes, particularly those in endurance or strength sports. However, it would be a mistake to say they are a small but representative sample of athletes. Almost without exception, these individuals are outstanding in their sport and also quite frequently are outstanding in other aspects of their lives. A few are considered the best athletes for their age group in their sport, nationally and internationally. And the many admirers of Bill Pearl and Frank Zane can make a convincing case that each one was the best *ever* in his sport.

All the athletes in this book were relatively easy to contact, gracious, and willing to take time out of their busy schedules to provide information for this book. The usual procedure involved an initial phone call where I briefly explained the overall purpose of the book. This was followed by a detailed letter that fully explained the book's scope and timetable and very detailed questionnaire. At this point, the athlete could choose to do the questionnaire alone, do long phone interviews in lieu of completing the questionnaire, or do some combination of both of these procedures. Most of the athletes opted to complete the questionnaire.

Phone interviews followed the questionnaire. Not surprisingly, because the interviews are interactive, the conversations often focused more on several key points, rather than the broader brush approach of the questionnaire. In some cases, phone interviews were used to clarify or broaden responses from the questionnaire.

A draft of the athlete's portrait was developed from these phone interviews and questionnaire responses. The draft was sent to the athlete for revision. In some cases, the draft and revision process was done up to four times to come up with a satisfactory portrait.

A total of 20 athletes were contacted in this way. Two female strength athletes and one female all-around athlete did not follow through with completing the questionnaire or requesting an interview. These figures (17 of 20) say to me that the overall approach was good, but probably my powers of persuasion with women leave something to be desired!

I attempted to contact five other athletes. Three were professional baseball players and two were professional (female) bodybuilders. In these cases, I could not talk with the athlete directly. Any phone or mail contact had to be directed through an agent, and no reply from the agent or athlete was ever received. Quite obviously, there is no substitute for direct personal contact.

Since the objective of the portraits was to do an in-depth study of a limited number of masters athletes and not a more superficial study of many athletes, I didn't make a concerted attempt to replace the athletes who declined to participate. I did, however, enlist the help of one of the featured athletes in contacting two female athletes.

PORTRAIT CONTENT

The content of the portraits focuses on the two major facets of this book: motivation and training. Of course, each portrait provides some background material about the athlete and tries to present some unique aspects of their lives. I also tried to encapsulate their individual philosophies by using a few of their own statements and to find out about any physical effects of aging.

As a research psychologist who has been trained over many years to be skeptical about data and qualify conclusions, I feel I must issue the proper caveats at this point. My original idea was actually to visit and observe each athlete train over a number of days. It quickly became apparent that financially and logistically that would not be possible. The questionnaire and phone interviews would have to suffice except for the few athletes who lived near me. I was able at times to informally see these athletes training and verify some information by talking with other people about the athlete.

So, for the most part, the athletes are telling us about their lives as they see them and in response to some particular questions. Many of us may reinterpret the past in light of present accomplishments. For example, we may see ourselves as being very purposeful in our youth when, perhaps, that was not all that true. And, specific types of questions tend to elicit specific kinds of responses. If you ask someone to detail their goals in life, do not be surprised when you sense them to be goal-directed individuals!

These caveats aside, I believe readers will be amazed at the relative consistency in these portraits. Over and over again, you will see reference to *focus, determination, personal standards and goal setting, planning and charting progress, and creating optimal environments*. These individuals bring to life the cognitive-social systems framework for behavior and motivation detailed in Chapter 2 and show the value of studying exemplar individuals. Recall that a good deal of study in psychology has been made of unmotivated people. Here, I take a more salutogenic approach.

At the same time, while many of these individuals are displaying high-level performance and striving over many years, quite a few seem to have a refreshingly adaptive perspective. While still achieving, and now often in more than one arena of life, many of the athletes have learned to "not take themselves so seriously," genuinely enjoy the process of achievement, and take time for other loving and relaxing pursuits.

After the portrait section, I will summarize more completely the common points found throughout the portraits. I will also pick out those points that appear unique and deserve particular attention. Later, I will take all these points, plus the major points from the chapters on motivation and behavior, periodization, and mental training and answer the question, "Well, what does all this mean for you?"

The athletes in the portrait section are either endurance (running, walking, swimming) or strength (bodybuilding, track and field) athletes. Since the emphasis is not on the uniqueness of the sport, but rather on motivation and training, the portraits are not presented by sport or by sex of the athlete. Indeed, after pondering what order would make the most sense, I have simply opted for alphabetical order.

CLARENCE BASS

Clarence Bass has achieved a lasting stature in the world of bodybuilding and Olympic lifting. As a teenager, over 30 years ago, he was one of the youngest and lightest men to clean and jerk 300 pounds. In his late 30s, Clarence turned to bodybuilding and soon was able to win his height class at the Mr. America Past 40 and Mr. USA Past 40 contests.

Clarence is known as "Mr. Ripped" in bodybuilding because he has consistently been able to reduce his body fat to below 3 percent. In fact, Clarence has been measured at the incredible level of 1 percent body fat! Most importantly, Clarence has demonstrated the nutritional and exercise methods that have kept his body fat percentage at a low level for many years.

Clarence is one of the most "defined" (the appearance of muscle separation and "cuts") bodybuilders of all time. However, Clarence was not always so lean. It took years of researching and experimenting with training and nutrition programs to achieve his goals.

Now, Clarence is one of the most creative and well-informed individuals in the world of bodybuilding and physical training. Moreover, beyond his specific accomplishments is found an approach to motivation and achievement that should be invaluable for many individuals in different walks of life.

At the age of 50, Clarence has achieved a high degree of success in five different parts of his life. First, he has been happily married to Carol since 1968, and they have a 15-year-old son, Matt. A life-long resident of Albuquerque, New Mexico, Clarence has over time built up a successful law practice, specializing in real estate. Every month, Clarence's "Ripped" column appears in *Muscle and Fitness,* a magazine with worldwide readership approaching two million. On his own, Clarence has written and marketed four excellent books on training and nutrition, the *Ripped* series and *The Lean Advantage.* The books are part of his extensive mail-order business. Finally, every year Clarence reaches a physical peak for pictures for his books and columns. Looking at the pictures, it is obvious that Clarence could step into any national level masters physique contest and continue to compete at the highest level. Of course, the question is "How did all of these accomplishments get started, and how are they continuing?"

Background and Approach

In Clarence's books and in an extremely sensitive recent column, Clarence credits his father, the late Hugh L. Bass, M.D., for his early and continued success. Hugh Bass was a terrific all-around athlete and, indeed, was literally a one-man track team, competing successfully in the pole vault, high jump, broad jump, and discus. Clarence was inspired by his example and admired the many medals he had won. At an early age, his father let Clarence use his weights and other equipment, but never pushed him to train or compete. When Clarence showed the interest, his father would take him to lifting meets,

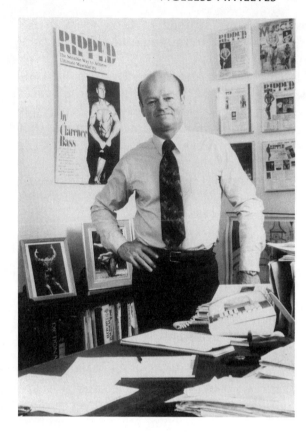

Clarence's law, business, and bodybuilding interests come together in his office.

and eventually his father equipped an exercise room suitable for training in Olympic lifting. But as Clarence has said, "Competing was always my idea, not his. He helped and encouraged me, but never pushed me."

As a high school student, Clarence also learned a lasting lesson. At that age, Clarence was small, in no way physically exceptional, and somewhat lacking in confidence in his own abilities. During his sophomore year, an upper-classmate was honored for winning the State High School Pentathlon Championship, which involved push-ups, chin-ups, jump reach, bar vault, and a 300-yard shuttle run. Years later Clarence noted, "Seeing that boy get his award as the whole school applauded inspired me. I made up my mind that I'd win that award the next year—and I did."

Besides the immediate reinforcement of the local paper's headline, "Bass is Strongest," Clarence learned a lifelong lesson and approach to success: Set hard but reachable goals, and channel your energies and talent to meet those goals. Clarence has been perceptive enough throughout his life to pick areas and goals where he has a clear sense that he can be successful. He found out at an early age that he enjoyed the process of working toward goals.

In fact, throughout his writings, Clarence emphasizes "enjoying the process" of working toward goals. His book, *Ripped-2*, ends with a quote from George Sheehan: "Happiness, we come to discover, is found in the pursuit of happiness."

More recently, in a book by Dominic Certo (*Success—Pure and Simple*, Keasbey, NJ: Hillside Publications, 1985, p. 125), Clarence has stated that: " . . . we all have strengths and weaknesses . . . it's important to decide what you do well and enjoy. Don't beat your head up against a wall trying to do something for which you aren't suited. Decide what you like to do and do best and then do it for all you're worth."

Besides his personal assessment and goal-setting strategy and approach, Clarence also found another key to motivation and success at an early age: control the setting and circumstances as much as possible. This perspective has been shown in many of Clarence's endeavors, from adopting a very early schedule in law school so he could study in peace and quiet at 4 A.M., a practice used more recently for training; to writing, producing, and marketing all his books himself; to establishing a private law practice in real estate and family law (after a successful career in a firm); to owning his own building to house his law practice, mail-order business, and his own private gym.

Current Sources of Motivation

As already suggested, Clarence's basic approach and goals have been lifelong and unfolding; his current accomplishments are not discontinuous with his past. His experiences in capturing his over-40 championships were not that different from his wins during his high school days. He attended national masters contests for two years prior to competing himself. He realized he had a good chance to win these contests and diligently went about working to accomplish that goal. His past history of goal setting and success provided the impetus to achieve a new goal. Or, as Clarence has said, "Success breeds success."

Clarence also quickly discovered that to maintain his magazine column (currently in its eighth year), he had to constantly search out new material. Further, he had to try out any new idea or method himself. This has kept the entire process—writing and training—fresh, interesting, and challenging.

Also, as noted, there are new pictures every year for his books and columns. Clarence typically sets a time of the year, often the late summer and early fall, to reach a peak for these photo sessions. And every year, he not only reaches a peak, but also he seems to have improved over the prior year. Thus, these year-end photo sessions take the place of peaking and training for competitions.

Clarence's personal standards in all his various activities remain to be the best he can possibly be by giving his best efforts. Training itself has been such an integral part of his life for so long that it is virtually impossible for Clarence to ever see himself stopping. His image of himself is someone who is healthy, fit, and strong. Clarence also noted that the appearance of his sedentary, professional peers, especially those in his age category, is enough impetus itself to keep training!

Thus, Clarence provides an excellent model to many individuals on how to be successful: choose the area you want to emphasize, pick reasonable goals, control as much as possible, and channel your energies. At the same time, he provides us with an important sense of balance: be sure you enjoy the process. For Clarence, "real winners" are people who steadily improve themselves and like what they are doing, not necessarily someone who walks away with a trophy.

At the same time, and by way of balance to his highly focused perspective, Clarence has reached another important conclusion: "I try not to take myself too seriously," he said.

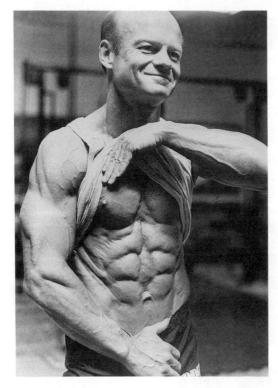

Clarence has some of the best "abs" in bodybuilding.

Training

Clarence's training has evolved over the years to the point where his approach is probably the most sophisticated in bodybuilding, and quite likely, more sophisticated than in other sports as well. The reason for this evolution is that Clarence is always eager to learn more about training and try out new ideas. This is not because of dissatisfaction, but rather because he finds trying different ways to train to be interesting, productive, efficient, and motivational.

Since Clarence's career spans Olympic lifting and bodybuilding over many years, it is safe to say that he has tried almost every known method of weight training. His lifting days were usually marked by four or five training sessions of about one and a half hours each per week. He usually emphasized using heavy weights for low repetitions, plus form and technique work.

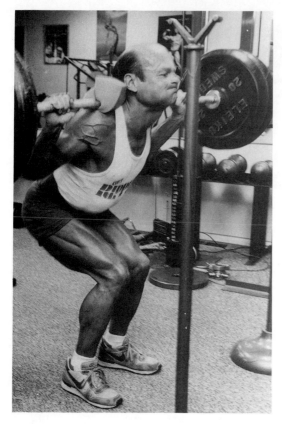

A former Olympic lifter, Clarence still emphasizes basic movements such as the squat in all his routines.

For bodybuilding, Clarence stayed with traditional routines—up to 20 sets per body part and as long as two hours a session—for only a short time. Like many of us, Clarence was struck by the message delivered in the 1970s by Arthur Jones, the developer of Nautilus, and Mike Mentzer, a Mr. Universe winner. Both emphasized basically the same idea: less was better, and the key to progress was intensity (i.e., heavy weights), training to failure, and use of negative and forced reps in short, focused sessions.

Clarence took this to heart and adapted the "super intensity" approach to his own training. This meant short sessions (less than an hour), training each body part twice every seven or eight days, and using high-intensity training methods. For a while, Clarence gained following these methods. However, he soon felt that he wasn't recovering sufficiently. His first solution started him down a very interesting road on a journey that continues today. Clarence differentiated between the first set of workouts for body parts, which were designed to be super intense, and a second go-around later in a week which were somewhat less intense. At first he only tried "straight sets," for example, no negative reps. He found that he still wasn't recovering that well. Next he tried using somewhat lighter weights for higher repetitions in his second set of workouts. Unfortunately, these workouts also could become quite hard.

Clarence's third step was borrowed mostly from the training of runners. Many years ago, runners adopted a hard day-easy day approach first advocated by Bill Bowerman at the University of Oregon. Clarence adapted this principle to bodybuilding by having the second set of workouts in a week use only 70–90 percent of the weight used for his intense workouts, while keeping to the same repetition scheme. The results were amazing. By only training intensely occasionally, he was able to make some outstanding gains in strength and muscle mass without experiencing breakdowns or sticking points that had characterized his super-intense approach.

This basic training schema was detailed in his book, *Ripped-2*, and undoubtedly has helped many individuals. However, Clarence was not content to rest on his laurels and the progress he had made in his own training. He sometimes found training to failure psychologically and physically very difficult. Clarence points out that training is supposed to be fun, not something to be dreaded. Frequent, super-intense sessions can become very draining and, indeed, counterproductive.

Clarence has recently been influenced by Fred Hatfield, who has emphasized using different rep schemes and performance modes to affect different cellular components of muscle, and Mike Stone and Harold O'Bryant, who have done extensive research and writing on the use of periodization in weight training. He also carefully studied and adapted Jan and Terry Todd's prescription for weight training (work a body part once per week at 100 percent and once at 85 percent) and their ideas on periodization. The general result has been the kind of program described in Chapter 3, and the specific results have shown in continued enthusiasm and gains for Clarence in his late 40s. Note that Clarence's approach is a creative adaptation and integration of the prior efforts by others and himself, and also emphasizes a good deal of variety.

Of course, the step-by-step goal setting and achievement that is at the core of periodization principles is also in tune with Clarence's overall motivational strategies. Periodization also emphasizes pushing hard and then backing off, a practice he has found works in other parts of his life. Thus, periodization fits Clarence almost perfectly.

Clarence has gone through a somewhat similar training evolution in his aerobic training, which will only be sketched here. This evolution has included periods in his younger days when he did virtually no aerobic training; some moderately successful efforts with running; extensive outdoor cycling that included long rides and hill charges; more moderate indoor cycling for shorter periods and for varying intensities; the use of an arsenal of aerobic equipment (ski machine, Air-Dyne, rower, bike, heavy hands) for about 45 minutes a day; and aerobic training that follows periodization principles and emphasizes the body parts worked on a given day with weights (e.g., accenting the arm part of the Air-Dyne when the upper body has been worked with weights), but which is clearly more moderate and secondary to weight training. Through reading and experimentation, Clarence has found an amount of aerobic training that satisfies health, metabolic, and calorie burning requirements, remains interesting, and does not undermine bodybuilding.

There are other parts of Clarence's training that are very instructive for masters athletes. Recently, Clarence has added a simple stretching routine that he performs *after* aerobic training. He has found that stretching helps prevent injury and speeds recovery. A mainstay for Clarence over many years has been walking. On his off days, he walks for about an hour, although the time may accumulate from two or three short sessions. On training days, he walks 15 to 20 minutes after lunch. All of Clarence's walking is done at a moderate pace. It is a time for thought, relaxation, and renewal and provides a balance for the stresses of work and training.

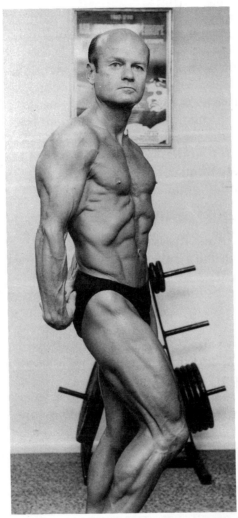

A great shot of Clarence at close to fifty.

Nutrition

As already noted, Clarence is one of the most "ripped" (defined) bodybuilders of all time and, perhaps, has achieved one of the lowest percentages of body fat of any adult athlete. Readers no doubt are wondering, "Does this man starve all the time or does he have some exotic, secret diet?" Neither is true. In actuality, Clarence has become an expert on nutrition, and his dietary guidelines closely follow those recommended by the National Cancer Institute and the American Heart Association.

In his recent book, *Ripped-3*, Clarence describes 22 of his favorite meals, including breakfasts, lunches, and dinners. All of these meals are easy to fix, and many use microwave cooking. A key to his meals is not only their simplicity and wholesomeness, but the fact that they are pleasant looking and tasting. Just as with training, good nutrition should be enjoyable.

The basic elements of Clarence's diet are now being accepted as fundamental elements of sound nutrition. These elements include:

- Eat whole foods the way they are grown. Unprocessed foods are usually low in calories but are tasty, chewy, and filling.
- Avoid calorie-dense and highly refined foods.
- Eat foods high in fiber such as grains, fruits, and vegetables.
- For protein sources, depend on low-fat milk products, nuts, beans, and occasionally fish, chicken, and eggs. Use beef only as a flavoring agent.

Thus, Clarence's diet is high in complex carbohydrates, low in fat, and moderate in protein. It is the kind of diet that is becoming a prescription for health, leanness, and athletic performance. And, as Clarence has noted, "It's a comfortable diet that makes you feel satisfied and never leaves you hungry. That's why it works so well" (*Ripped-3*, p. 19).

It should be noted that Clarence does supplement his basic diet, although *not* to the extent of other athletes. Clarence's supplements usually include a good multivitamin/mineral plus moderate dosages of vitamins B, C, and E. Basically, Clarence feels that an athlete can reach the very top by just following a simple, healthful diet.

Postscript

Since Clarence achieved so much in his 30s and 40s, and has just reached 50, I was curious to know what Clarence's goals and plans were for this, the sixth, decade of his life. He says he isn't sure. The recent death of his father has resulted in more family responsibilities and his law practice has grown markedly as well. He simply has not had time for long-range planning. But stay tuned. You can be sure that whatever Clarence decides to do, he will do it his way, for all that he's worth, while remembering to keep things in perspective and enjoyable.

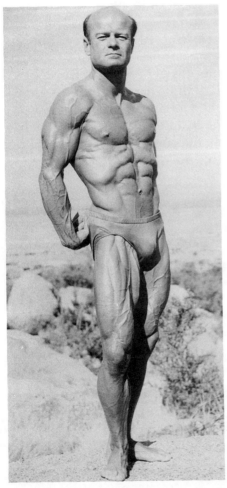

A combination of bodybuilding, aerobics, and proper nutrition leads to Clarence's incredibly ripped appearance.

BARRY BROWN

Since Barry Brown's advanced degree is a Juris Doctorate, it appears appropriate to say that irrefutable evidence can be presented that he is the best masters runner in the country, and quite possibly the world. His list of accomplishments, as we will see shortly, is astonishing, and his longevity at the top of the field is simply incomparable. But perhaps more heartening for other masters athletes is that Barry Brown is still improving in longer distances.

Barry was born in July 1944, in Albany, New York. He graduated from Colonie Central High School in 1962. In 1966 Barry received a degree in business from Providence College, and the aforementioned law degree from Albany Law School in 1969.

Currently, Barry resides six months of the year in Florida and six months in New York. This unique arrangement is made possible by having an office and home in both Gainesville, Florida, and Glens Falls, New York. In each location, Barry has a separate set of clients. During the summer, Barry commutes back to Florida once per month, and in the winter he is in New

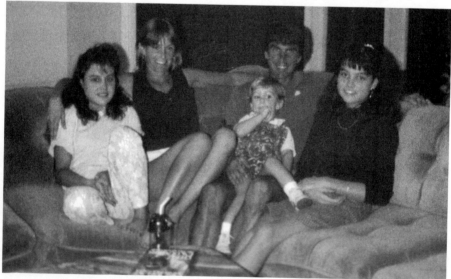

The Brown family: Candy, Bobbi, Darren, Barry, and Stacy

York twice per month. Barry owns his own firm, Equity Planning Services, Inc. and, besides managerial responsibilities, consults on retirement plans and fringe benefits.

Barry married Bobbi in December 1984. He has two children—Stacy, 17, and Candy, 16—by a previous marriage, and a son, Darren, 2, with Bobbi. Bobbi is also a serious competitive runner, logging 50–70 miles per week. She is capable of running the 10K in about 38 minutes.

Accomplishments

Barry has been training consistently for over 30 years. In high school, he focused on the one-mile run, and in college ran the mile and two-mile runs. From the time he was 23 until he was 36, Barry specialized in the steeplechase. By his mid-30s, his repertoire had broadened to include 10Ks, 15Ks, half-marathons, and marathons.

And now the list of Barry's accomplishments:

- Barry has represented the United States in 23 international competitions.
- Barry qualified for the 1968, 1972, 1976, and 1980 Olympic Trials.
- Barry ran a sub-four-minute mile in 1973.
- Barry was the RRCA (Road Runners Club of America) masters runner of the year in 1984, 1985, and 1986.
- Barry has held the U.S. Masters-records for the 3K, 8K, 10K, 10-mile, 20K, half-marathon, 20-mile, and marathon.

Training

Barry's accomplishments are indeed astonishing. But Barry insists that he is not particularly gifted or naturally talented. For example, Barry feels that his leg speed is actually on the slow side. Instead, his accomplishments are a tribute to his perseverance, discipline, and, of course, motivation. In other words, here is a champion who "was made, not born."

Barry trains twice a day, virtually every day, at 7 A.M. and 4:30 P.M. He consistently totals 120–150 miles per week; that's between about 17 and 20 miles per day! Barry has tried lower mileage regimes, but his performance in races told him that lower volume did not work for him. Upping his mileage led again to better performance.

If Barry has made a concession to age, it's in the frequency of high-intensity workouts. He does these workouts twice per week, while 10–15 years ago he did them three times per week, and when he was in his 20s, four times per week. Barry's experience substantiates the conclusion we made in Chapter 3, that within reason, the frequency of hard workouts may not matter so much. What is important for top performance is that hard workouts are consistently done at a high intensity.

Barry's training includes two interval sessions, one with shorter repetitions and one with longer repetitions. Both workouts take about 90 minutes to complete including a warm-up and cool-down, with the high-intensity part lasting between 30–45 minutes.

An example of a shorter repetition workout is:

4 × 400 in 65 seconds with a 200 jog
3 × 150 in a relaxed, moderately fast pace with a 150 jog
4 × 400 in 65 seconds with a 200 jog
3 × 150 in a relaxed, moderately fast pace with a 150 jog
5 × 200 in 30–32 seconds with a 200 jog.

A longer repetition workout can be:

7 × 1 mile in 4:50 to 4:40 with a 400 interval, or
10 × 800 in 2:16 to 2:20 with a 400 interval.

It is apparent that these are ultraserious workouts. An example of a typical week's schedule is shown in Table 1.

Barry has a simple method for conceding as little as possible to aging in training—don't stop. However, realistically and intelligently, Barry has made some adaptations to age. As Barry's schedule shows, an intense workout is now followed by two

TABLE 1

TYPICAL TRAINING WEEK FOR BARRY BROWN

Day	A.M.	Pace	P.M.	Pace
Monday	7–8 miles	6:30	10 miles	6:15–7:00
Tuesday	7–8 miles	6:30	Intervals 10–12 miles	
Wednesday	7–8 miles	6:30	15	6:00–6:30
Thursday	7–8 miles	6:30	10	6:15–7:00
Friday	7–8 miles	6:30	Intervals 10–12 miles	
Saturday	15	6:15–6:30	7–8	Easy
Sunday	17–20	6:15–6:30	8	Easy

Weekly Total = 137–150 miles

easier days. Barry also reported that now he feels joint stiffness in the morning, some lack of flexibility, and that his potential for injury is higher than before. Barry has incorporated stretching and weight training with light weights and high repetitions in his routine. He tries to run more on soft surfaces and, except for races, avoids all-out sprints.

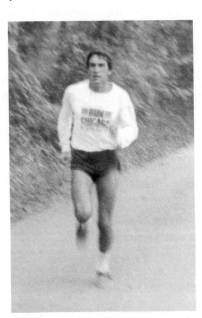

Barry on a relaxed training run shows terrific form.

Despite this well-rounded and thoughtful approach, Barry did suffer the first serious injury of his career in April 1985, a chronically sprained deltoid ligament in his left ankle. He now wears more supportive running shoes and avoids running on cambered roads. However, to put the injury into perspective, Barry can still do training runs of 20 miles and race for 13 miles (5:00 to 5:15 pace) without pain as long as he wears the right shoes and stays away from cambered roads.

Perhaps more than any other athlete featured in this book, the answer to the question, "What keeps Barry training and performing at such a super level?" is found in the unique interplay of beliefs, emotions, behavior, and environmental influences. It is instructive to delineate these elements separately and then examine how they interact following the model discussed in detail in Chapter 2.

Personal Progress

Self-Standards   Barry's personal standards for excellence are both highly specific and incredibly lofty, though not unrealistic. They include running 120–150 miles per week, winning all the masters races he runs, placing high in the open division, and holding all masters records for the mile through marathon. Barry's goals for performance are based on his personal best 15 years ago. He may be slightly slower at shorter distances, but he is now equal to or better than his youthful self at longer distances. His personal standards, however, keep evolving because he keeps improving and what he feels is possible keeps ascending. Because he is the best at what he does, Barry's response to questions about his standards is unique. He wrote that he wants to "run much faster than any 40-year-old has considered running" and "completely redefine what a 40-year-old is capable of."

Self-Observation   Barry tracks his performance and training on a daily basis. He keeps a detailed log where he records the miles he ran, the time, the effort put into the workout, his energy level, and any aches and pains. He is thus capable of comparing workouts across an extended time frame. He also measures himself against particular training partners (although he most often trains alone), and he competes quite often.

Self-Evaluation and Affect   Matching or exceeding personal standards is very important to Barry, and being successful leads to more self-confidence, what we've called in this book *self-efficacy*. Failure to meet goals and standards disappoints Barry, but through self-analyses, it also leads him to change his training and effort to make sure he meets his goals the next time. So Barry is unlikely to become very depressed about a disappointing performance. While Barry finds reaching goals and standards satisfying, he doesn't use tangible rewards since, as he notes, "You're only as good as your last race." Thus, in many respects, Barry has learned to realistically temper his moods, never reaching the depths of depression reported by some athletes.

In summary, Barry's personal processes of motivation center on having extremely high personal standards and setting up specialized training and monitoring systems to meet those standards, which have resulted in high outcome expectancies and self-efficacy. Not surprisingly, these standards and beliefs exert influence on the environment which, in turn, Barry tries to arrange to enhance high motivation and training.

General and External Influences

Almost 20 years ago, at an age when many former college athletes are retiring from serious competition, Barry made an eventful decision: to live in Florida for most of the year so that the weather would be optimal for training. As noted, Barry has developed his business so that it is possible to divide his time between New York and Florida, thus taking advantage of the best weather in the North and South.

The business that he has set up also provides the flexibility for his daily training schedule and geographic mobility. Time with his family and other daily activities also revolve around this training schedule. Thus, the different parts of Barry's life fit together and seem to enhance each other.

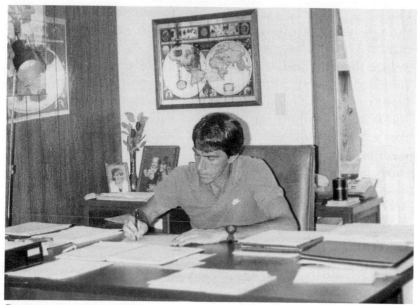

Barry at one of the sites of his successful planning and investment agency.

Outcome Expectancies   As noted above, over time and through trial and error, Barry's program has evolved to its present form—high mileage, twice per day running, plus two hard interval sessions per week. Experiments with other programs simply have not worked for him. By careful observation, Barry has found that his best times come from his present program and his best races are run after three to six weeks of high mileage followed by a short tapering off period. Thus, at this point, Barry's confidence in his program is very high.

Self-Efficacy   Unlike some outstanding masters athletes, Barry's belief in his own abilities is not based on his belief in genetic superiority. Rather, the basis for Barry's belief in his abilities rests on his ascending performance over many years and his perseverance. This translates into a willingness to work very hard over a long period of time to develop the abilities that he does have to their ultimate form. For example, Barry noted that "I'm not very talented compared to most and my leg speed is terrible, but I have developed my strength and endurance" (i.e., a 4:28 mile in 1962 to 3:58 in 1973).

Critical Enactive Behaviors

Besides structuring his environment to allow for optimal training, Barry uses several key behaviors to increase his motivation and enhance his training and racing.

Preparation for Hard Training Sessions   As described above, Barry's hard training sessions are well-planned and extremely intense. He often spends two or three days prior to a hard workout convincing himself that it is "doable." One method he employs is to break down the workout into segments and concentrate on (visualize) optimal performance in each segment. Such preparation seems necessary because these sessions are so intense and because he usually trains alone. There is no one else to set a pace or provide other sources of help and motivation.

Preparation for Races   Barry cautions that for racing, there is no substitute for hard training. However, for several days preceding a race, Barry employs visualization and imagery techniques. He imagines that he can relax while running at race pace. A day or two before competition, Barry will run a few 200s or 400s at race pace to show himself how easy it is. Note how well these techniques fit the notion of reciprocity between cognitions and behaviors. Visualization and imagery prepare him for hard training sessions and optimal race performance. Intense training and his preparation allow him to sample race pace before a competition. The ease of the sample race pace fuels self-efficacy beliefs and the cognitive preparation strategies.

Critical External Influences

Goals   Competition, winning races, setting records, and personal bests are the major motivations for Barry. Everything in his training is geared toward maximum performance and achieving goals. Since reaching 40, Barry has had new goals to achieve. This is probably the reason that, compared to his 20s and 30s, his motivation now for training and competition is "much higher."

Other Influences　　Barry's wife, Bobbi, is very supportive of his efforts. She provides feedback about his training and performance and is in general a moderating influence in his life. However, Barry is entirely self-coached (for over 20 years), does not have training partners, does not socialize only with other runners, and does not belong to an athletic organization. Years ago, Jack Bacheler (currently a well-known coach at North Carolina State) was a role model in that he showed Barry how to train consistently and effectively. However, at this point, in a real sense, Barry is his own role model. Specialized magazines provide some source of motivation because they give Barry new training ideas and occasionally feature other masters runners. As for financial returns, lest anyone believe that masters road racing is lined with gold, Barry noted that he could probably earn more money by not racing and spending more time on his business. Thus, out of an array of potential external motivational influences, goals and goal setting seem to be most important for Barry.

Commitment and Feedback　　Barry directly relates commitment and feedback to specific goals. Barry has told his wife, occasional training partners, and members of the media that on good racing days he will run a sub-4:10 mile and break Jack Foster's Masters Marathon record (2: 11:19). Bobbi is capable of providing pinpoint feedback about his training and performance, and Barry's training logs provide favorable feedback. Barry gets social reinforcement for his efforts from the approval of Barry's children and training partners who often express awe at his workouts and his races. In general, reactions of younger people to Barry have been mixed. They respect him for his achievements, but resent being beaten by him. Barry, in turn, has become more determined to beat his younger rivals. To some middle-aged people, Barry is becoming a "middle-aged hero." People his own age are very supportive, are often incredulous about his performance, and look to him as an inspiration to accomplish more in their own athletic lives. Coupled with his public commitments, the reactions of peers provide fertile ground for motivation but also exact the price of obligation and dedication from Barry.

Conclusions

The answers to the questions "What makes a champion?" and "What keeps a person performing at such an incredibly high level for so long?" are not simple ones. We see in Barry's portrait an almost perfect blending of a variety of internal and external factors whose interplay is a starting point to answer those questions. These points can be briefly summarized:

1. *Environmental:* Barry has structured and arranged his personal and professional life to maximize training and performance. He receives support and positive feedback from a few close and respected individuals. Goal attainment, such as winning races and setting masters records, is extremely important to Barry.

2. *Behaviors:* Through long experience, Barry has evolved a training program that has the right mix of frequency, intensity, and volume for him. He has been able through keen observations to fine-tune the schedule (e.g., changes in surface, reduction in the frequency of interval sessions) and also to adopt particular techniques (e.g., visualization) to maximize hard training sessions.

3. *Beliefs and Cognitions:* Barry's personal standards are extremely lofty, yet specific and realistic. Because these standards are realistic, performances can match or exceed standards. Therefore, self-efficacy and outcome expectancies remain high.

4. *Affect:* Barry's emotional responses to the ups and downs of training and competing stay very appropriate. He keeps good and poor performances in perspective, reacts to them, and analyzes them, making relevant changes in beliefs, behaviors, or the environment.

BEVERLY CROWN

Background

For many of the athletes featured in this book, success started at an early age, and one success led to others. These individuals appear to have learned invaluable lessons, often in their teens, about picking goals and channelling their time and energy to meet those goals. Beverly Crown, on the other hand, has had a different and fascinating route to her current life as a successful businesswoman and one of the top masters bodybuilders in the country.

Beverly feels that she has lived two separate lives. In her first life, Beverly, who was born in August 1939 in Gary, Indiana, followed traditional role expectations for a girl from a devout Catholic family. Although a good student in high school, her college career was abruptly ended at 18. Beverly married her former high school teacher and, after one year of marriage, was pregnant. Eventually, Beverly would have three children— Debra, now 29; Tawne, 26; and Lance, 23.

By the time she was in her early 20s, Beverly knew she needed to get out of the confines of a traditional marriage. An acute need eventually propelled her into her second life: the family was poor and desperately needed money. Living around the Chicago area, Beverly came up with the quickest way she could think of to make decent money. In 1962, she became a Playboy Bunny!

Beverly explained that it was only in this job that she felt her drive, intensity, and good looks could propel her into a better life. It was at that point that she understood a philosophy that her father, an American Indian, tried to give Beverly: "Always make the best possible use of what (resources, attributes) you have."

A few years after her start at the Playboy Club, Beverly met her second husband, Barry Crown, who is from a wealthy business family. To look at her now, you would think that Beverly's "second life" has been easy and successful. After all, she helped develop a small firm, Henderson Camp Products, into a major company in the field in just 11 years. She has run marathons and come in in second place in a national open AAU couples bodybuilding competition. Her marriage remains happy and fulfilling, and she is in demand for a variety of community, business, and charitable activities.

What is less apparent is that Beverly has reached some of the

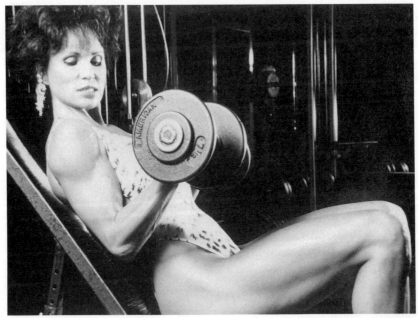

Beverly shows that fitness and beauty go hand-in-hand in the middle years.

most incredible highs and lows of any individual. Her life has been "a series of obstacles" and, at several times, an absolute "struggle to live."

During a 10-year period, Beverly had five major surgeries: double kidney operations, double lung operations, and a back operation. The back injury was the result of an automobile accident. Through some atypical responses to anesthesia, Beverly was partly awake during her operations. She had incredible "out of body" experiences and was able to virtually watch herself being operated on. Even more frightening, a number of times she almost died on the operating table or in the hospital.

At best, recovery from a serious operation can take a year to 18 months. When serious operations come one after another, recovery takes longer and is more tenuous. Thus, it is remarkable that Beverly is as fit and active as she is today.

These experiences and struggles have given Beverly the strong beliefs that she must "plug into the most positive energy" and "appreciate and maximize every moment." Her daily life is an affirmation of her ability to overcome any obstacles placed in her way, and particular moments, such as appearing on stage in a bodybuilding show, are an absolute triumph.

Although Beverly is well-off financially, these experiences have led her to a firm belief—no mere platitude for her—that "good health is the most valuable possession anyone can have," and "you really know that when you're losing it."

Throughout her physical ordeals and her remarkable recoveries, Beverly was sustained by a never-ending belief in her ability to prevail and a "glimmer inside of her" that signified that her physical being was on the mend. These beliefs and feelings parallel Dr. Aaron Antonovsky's concept of a "sense of coherence"—a sense that life and events eventually work out for the best for you—which he sees as central to health maintenance.

Beverly's general motto for living is clear: "As long as you have life, you can do anything!"

Training, Athletics, and Aging

It should not be surprising that Beverly came to fitness and bodybuilding activities through no ordinary route. In the early 1980s Beverly and Barry met Sir Edmund Hillary, the legendary mountain climber. They were persuaded to take a trip to Mount Everest. Although Beverly had always done some aerobic training because of a history of heart disease in her family, the training for the mountain trip, which included running and Nautilus machines, was more rigorous. For a month, Beverly lived on the mountain at the 18,000-foot base camp, making daily climbs. This experience gave Beverly much more of a sense of her physical self, her physical potential, and her responsibility to care for and develop her body, and it launched her into a commitment to fitness and bodybuilding. Barry, in turn, has become a marathon runner.

Beverly is quick to point out that in bodybuilding she is struggling to overcome limitations. For example, virtually every bodybuilder, male or female, will say that you cannot really become good without doing heavy barbell squatting at least some time in your career. Because of Beverly's back injury and other operations, squatting is not possible. She has to work around her limitations and just push on.

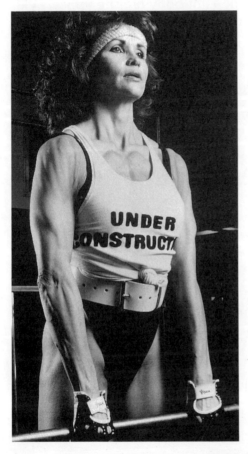

Beverly relies on many basic movements in her routines.

Incidentally, Beverly feels it was the discipline and physical condition she achieved through bodybuilding that enabled her to come back after her back operation for a crushed disc. Her doctors were amazed at her recovery ability, although no one predicted she could return to top-level bodybuilding.

In addition, very few people believed that a woman just

starting bodybuilding in her 40s could make impressive gains. Beverly has shown it can be done. She has gained about 10 pounds since she started and appreciably lowered her body fat percentage. Again, this is a good example of making use of your best attributes. Beverly is not very large or powerful, but at between 12–13 percent body fat, she appears extremely fit and athletic—which, of course, she is.

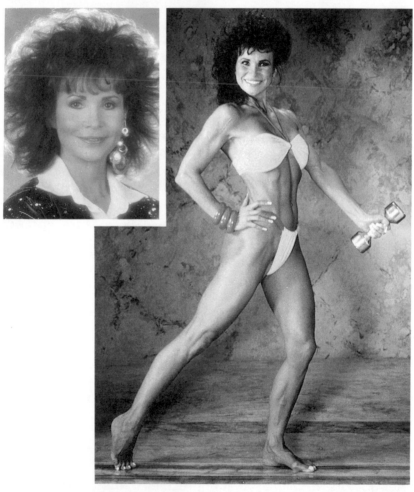

It's hard to believe that Beverly is almost fifty. It is even harder to believe that in recent years she has had five major operations.

Beverly believes that middle-aged athletes in particular, who are naturally atrophying at this point in their lives, have to be extremely careful with nutrition. Her very low-fat, high protein (lean), and high-complex carbohydrate diet is further enriched with multivitamins and protein supplements.

Beverly's daily schedule, which has been cut back because she is still recovering from her back surgery, is similar to many of the schedules of other masters athletes in this book. She and Barry get up each day between 5:00 and 6:00 A.M. After coffee, a snack, and vitamins, Beverly runs or does indoor cycling for from 30 to 60 minutes. After breakfast, she attends to business matters and then to her community responsibilities.

In the late afternoon, she usually weight trains at a gym and does additional aerobics, for a total training time of up to two hours. She averages about an hour a day of aerobic activity.

Evenings often include dining out and simple, quiet, and relaxing time at home. Even when the Crowns travel, which can be about a third of each year, Beverly likes to keep a similar schedule.

Most impressively, despite a 15 percent loss of lung capacity through her operations, Beverly has scored in the "excellent" range, just a hair short of "superior," when tested at the Cooper Clinic in Dallas. Beverly believes that the superior rating is within her grasp.

Beverly is also seriously considering a return to bodybuilding competition. Recently, her training has been going well, and she says she can feel a new surge of power. What she has in mind is sensible, hard training for the next two years and entering masters contests at the age of 50 as a birthday present to herself.

Realistically, Beverly feels that she probably will not win. Many female competitors are much more muscular than they were even a few years ago. However, going through the entire process, she feels, will be challenging and rewarding. By simply being able to compete, she will be a winner.

Beverly does not see herself stopping training at any point. She notes, "Since I started, I have never thought about discontinuing training. At this point, it's my way of life."

Beverly also believes that in many ways aging has been mis-represented. She has a much more functional definition of age: "Age is nothing more than the inability to do what you did when you were younger." In a sense, if you can do more than when you were younger, you are not aging. Thus, through her business, community, fitness, and bodybuilding activities, Beverly is helping to redefine "aging."

Beverly is thinking about returning to competition when she is fifty!

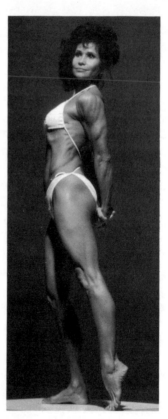

What are her goals for the future? A return to top physical shape has already been noted. As Beverly continues to recover, she also wants to devote more time to her business and community activities. She would also like to take another trip to an isolated spot in the world and become rejuvenated through an intensely physical and spiritual experience. She sees adopting a simpler, almost "back to nature," life-style at some later point. Ranching may be her choice sometime in the future.

Most of all, Beverly would like to achieve a different kind of success. This type is differentiated from fame and from the day-to-day success that she strives for in all aspects of her life. Real success for Beverly means being able to make contributions to people and the community on a consistent, daily basis. That is what she is striving for, and she will undoubtedly achieve it.

BARBARA FILUTZE

Twelve years ago, at the age of 30, Barbara Filutze started to get concerned about her health, fitness, and physical conditioning. She was smoking 30 cigarettes a day at the time. Barb learned to play tennis and racquetball and enjoyed local league competition. But she still continued to smoke.

It seemed to Barb that a more strenuous activity that was incompatible with smoking would help her kick addiction to nicotine. The rest of her family was already competing in running, so Barb decided to become a runner. Although Barb was smoking a cigarette at the starting line, she managed to win a three-mile "fun run" race with a time of 21 minutes, and a competitive spirit was born.

There is little doubt that today Barb is the top female Masters long-distance runner in the country. Indeed, Barb is reasonably competitive at an international level in *open* meets!

Background

Barb was born in June 1946 in Erie, Pennsylvania, where she still lives. She completed high school at the Villa Maria Academy, an all-girls' school, where she was a good student but participated in no sports. Basketball was the only team sport at that time, and Barb was not allowed to join the team.

Barbara married Michael in 1966, and they have three children: Lisa, 20; Geoffrey, 17; and Erin, 12. While the children were young, Barb did not work outside the home and devoted herself to her family and home. Today, she works part-time as a bank teller and as a cross-country and long-distance track coach at a prep school. She also contributes to her family's income through the prize money she earns racing.

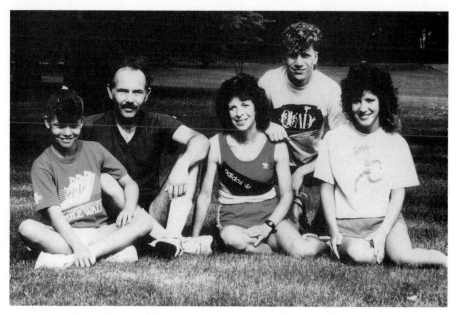

The Filutze family: Erin, Michael, Barb, Geoffrey, and Lisa.

Because Barbara provided considerable detail in completing her questionnaire, her coming of age as an athlete can be chronicled as shown in Table 2.

TABLE 2

Year	Age	Activity	Training	Nutrition
1976	30	Tennis	Lessons 5 days a week League play 1 day	Reduced red meat
1977	31	Racquetball	League play 2 days a week Tennis 1 day a week	Reduced fat in diet
1978	32	Running	Tried to run every day, but only ran 181 miles that year; ran 3 races; 54:40 for 10K	Continued to reduce fat
1979	33	Running	Ran 1,665 miles and 20 races; 38:43 for 10K and 3:15:56 for marathon	Same
1980	34	Running	Ran 2,327 miles and 22 races; 39:16 for 10K and 3:13:33 for marathon	Same
1981	35	Running	Ran 2,405 miles and 21 races; 36:24 for 10K and 2:55:45 for marathon	Same
1982	36	Running	Ran 3,316 miles and 24 races; 35:05 for 10K (U.S. rècord) and 2:46:36 for marathon	Almost a vegetarian
1983	37	Running	Ran 2,600 miles and 17 races; 35:04 for 10K and 2:44:16 marathon; set U.S. record for 25K (1:35:07); qualified for 1st Women's Olympic Trials	Same
1984	38	Running	Ran 3,600 miles and 24 races; 33:36 for 10K and 2:41:18 for marathon; set U.S. single-age records for 10 miles (59:08), 10K (33:36, a 35–39 age group record); and marathon (2:41:18); participated in Olympic Trials (2:43:45, 58th place)	Same
1985	39	Running	Ran 3,609 miles and 21 races; 34:04 for 10K and 2:45:06 for marathon; set U.S. single-age records for 10 miles (58:32) ½ marathon (1:16:44), 10K (34:04), and 5K (17:50)	Same

TABLE 2 continued

Year	Age	Activity	Training	Nutrition
1986	40	Running	Ran 3,096 miles and 24 races; 34:31 for 10K and 2:42:38 for marathon; set U.S. masters records for 5K (17:25), ½ marathon (1:16:00); qualified for Olympic Trials at 3 marathons. Voted "Outstanding Athlete 1986" for females 40–44 by TAC, the Athletics Congress.	
1987	41	Running	Ran 3,275 miles and 22 races; 33:41 for 10K and 2:42:48 for marathon; competed as first master for U.S. Open team at World Cup Marathon in Seoul, South Korea on '88 Olympic Marathon course; broke own U.S. masters record for 5K in 16:58:5 (P.R.); masters winner at Los Angeles Marathon, Pittsburgh Marathon, Legg's Mini-Marathon, Asbury Park 10K Classic, Maggie Valley 5 Miler, Albany National Masters 10K, and Great Race 10K, setting new masters 10K record	Same

Goals, Accomplishments, and Training Program

Table 2 shows that, while Barb has not been training for as many years as most of the masters athletes in this book, her training over the last nine years has been both rigorous and consistent. Her biggest breakthroughs in performance occurred after about five years of training. Since that time, inch by inch and second by second, Barb has steadfastly improved.

From 1979 to 1986, Barb's major goals were to train and race at all distances from the 5K to the marathon. When she was well prepared, Barbara would try for PRs in her races. Her more specific goals were to qualify for the Olympic Marathon Trials in 1984 and 1988. Barb also wanted to set masters records from the 5K to the marathon and to be ranked as the number one women's masters runner in the country.

Barb's goals have been lofty, but realistic. She qualified and competed in the first women's Olympic marathon trial in 1984 and took 58th place with a PR of 2:43:45. She easily qualified for the 1988 trials. Of course, keep in mind that these were open competitions.

Since age 36, Barb has set 15 U.S. women's records, including the masters records in the half-marathon (1:16:00) and twice for 5K (17:25 and 16:58) and 10K (33:41). Barb also became the first masters athlete, male or female, to compete internationally for the United States when she ran the World Cup Marathon in Seoul, South Korea (in April 1987). However, Barb is particularly proud of a more personal record. She has started and completed 38 marathons without walking, and she completed all but a few in under three hours.

Possibly because Barb only started serious training in her 30s, or perhaps because of constitutional factors, Barb reports no noticeable physical effects of aging. Her performances are still improving, and Barb indicated that she feels better and can train harder than she could when in her early 30s.

By most standards for internationally ranked runners, Barb's training program is decidedly modest and "sane." She averages about 70 miles per week. When she has a weekend race, her schedule consists of one track workout with only several really hard miles, one long run of 15 or more miles, and several easier days. If she does not have a race, her schedule may include two track workouts, or one track workout and a road workout (e.g., one mile repeats in a fartlek workout), the long run, and the several days of easier running. Most of her training is done in the late afternoons with the long run done Sunday morning. Examples of Barb's workouts are shown in Table 3 (p. 136).

Barb works out under the guidance of her husband, who formulates a weekly schedule, and also works with two coaches. Bill Hoffman is a track coach, and Doug Watts of Edinboro College works with Barb on track and road workouts. Barb does some road workouts alone. As the table shows, Barb's hard workouts are, indeed, very hard. She has learned to build up slowly over the year and take easy days, an approach similar to the one described in Chapter 3.

TABLE 3

EXAMPLES OF BARBARA FILUTZE'S WORKOUTS*

Coach Hoffman	Coach Watts		Alone
Track	Track	Road	Track & Road
1. 5 × ½ mile, 2:34, 2:35, 2:34, 2:33, 2:33; 2 × ¼ mile, :72, :72	1. 1,200 meters, 4:12; 1,200 meters, 4:07; 800 meters, 2:39	1. 7-mile hill run in 43:07, 1st mile in 5:22	1. 7.5 mile hill timed workout, 45:39
2. 4 × 1 mile, 5:19, 5:50, 5:19, 5:50	2. 8 × ½ mile repeats in 2:39 to 2:41 with a 2-minute interval	2. ½ marathon time trial in 1:19:53, on hills	2. 3 × ⅓ mile hill repeats; 2 × ½ mile; 2 × ½ mile, downhill
3. 4 × 1,200 meters, 3:56, 3:58, 4:00, 4:02	3. 1,500 meters, 5:07; 1,000 meters, 3:13; 1,000 meters, 3:16; 1,500 meters, 5:05	3. 3 × 2 miles on dirt roads, 11:27, 10:59, 11:18	3. 2 sets of 2 hills, 3 × ¼ mile, 1 × ⅓ mile downhill
4. 6 × ½ mile, 2:41, 2:36, 2:36, 2:36; 1 × 200 meters, 2 × 400 meters, 1 × 200 meters	4. 8 × ¼ mile, :70 to :73	4. 2 miles in 11:13; 3 miles in 17:15; 4 × 200 meters on track and striders	4. 9 × ¼ mile 9 × 150 meters
5. 12 × ¼ mile, :73, :73, :73, :73, :72, :74, :74, :74, :74, :74, :74, :74	5. 3,000 meters, 10:36, 1,500 meters, 5:09; 3,000 meters, 10:47		5. Fartlek long run with repeats of 6, 5, 4, 3, 2, 1 minutes and rests of half the time
6. 400 meters, 1:19; 800 meters, 2:40; 1,200 meters, 4:01; 1,600 meters, 5:21; 1,200 meters, 4:03; 800 meters, 2:39; 400 meters, 1:16			

*Barb always tries to do slightly better than time goals for workouts.

Barb picking up the pace in
an early fall training run.

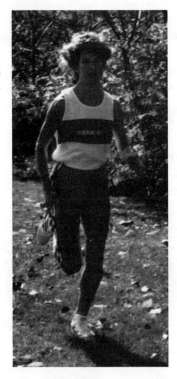

This schedule represents a recent change in her approach. Barb feels that her focus on speed, which was usually confined to 10 weeks in the summer with friend and coach Bill Hoffman, was not enough. Starting in 1987, Barb asked Coach Watts to let her come and work out with his other runners once or twice a week, early spring through late fall, alternating workouts with Coach Hoffman during the summer months.

Barb has a very tough approach to her training that is best expressed in her own words:

> I follow my weekly schedule to the "T" and never back down on the number of miles or the amount of the workout. I really feel this helps deter a breakdown during a race.

However, Barb has not been without injuries. About every two years, she has had a serious injury. For example, in 1986, a hamstring injury sidelined her for three months. From time to time she has experienced some knee problems. She has experimented with different shoes, training surfaces, and workouts to alleviate injuries.

Motivation: External Factors

Barb credits her husband Michael for helping her lay out and reach her goals. Mike provides Barb with considerable social support, serves as her coach and sometime training partner, drives her to races, and is her companion on trips. Indeed, all members of the family are runners, creating a unique bond in the family.

Barb and daughter Lisa.

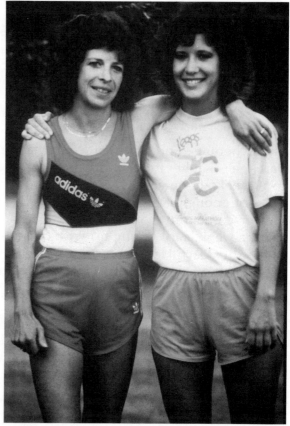

At the beginning of the year, during their long winter runs, Barb and Mike formulate particular goals, races, and training plans for the year. For example, in 1987, Barb's overall goal was to be the number one female masters runner in the country. Subgoals included competing locally in open competition and winning all her races. Barb explained that once these goals are set and the winter ends, "I simply work toward these goals until my rest period, Thanksgiving until New Year's."

Barb sometimes trains with a number of male friends who can help her keep a good pace, and she is fortunate to work with two well-known and respected coaches. Earning prize money is important and motivating, but Barb feels that she will only receive financial returns for a few years. She admits that some of the younger women coming up may have more speed than she will have by then.

It is only recently that Barb has received attention in *Sports Illustrated*, running magazines, and local newspapers. She welcomes such attention, but she doesn't need it for her athletic development. Barb has had an important role model, however. She has been able to emulate Priscilla Welch, who has held many world masters records and was the first female finisher in the 1987 New York Marathon. Barb feels that despite Priscilla's competitiveness, she is very humble and down to earth and always takes the time to encourage other runners. Barb credits Priscilla with giving her the simplest and best advice for running. Before a 1985 marathon, Priscilla said, "Give it all you've got."

To guide her training and racing efforts, Barb keeps a very detailed log. Her records include a detailed description of her workouts, cumulative weekly and monthly mileage, race splits, times, and female and overall position, all in juxtaposition to her goals. Barb also uses a public commitment strategy to help keep her motivated. However, rather than predicting what she will do in an upcoming race, Barb will say what she would *like* to do. She takes great satisfaction in meeting these commitments.

Not surprisingly, Barb is always "up" for her competitions, even minor ones. She always has being the first female finisher as her goal, and she really enjoys coming in before younger women. These feelings contrast with how she feels prior to many workouts:

> I am never "up" for a workout. Just before starting, I always have some excuse—"not feeling well," "tired," "legs not ready," "too sore." But after the warmup and striders and the first 400 meters, I feel better and actually get stronger as the workout progresses. I think of my goals when I'm getting tired.

Barb, like a number of other masters athletes (e.g., Joe Germana), has found one simple solution for overcoming "training blahs": just start the workout and focus on your goals. Barb credits the support of her husband, coaches, and running peers for keeping her motivated over the long haul. Younger people, amazed with her training and racing performance, are particularly supportive. Reactions from peers of her own age have been mixed: some wonder out loud when Barb will stop.

Although Barb works only part-time outside the home, her training environment is less than ideal when compared to other world-class athletes. She must fit her workouts in between work, family, and home responsibilities. And she trains through the long, cold Pennsylvania winters (although this may help her in the long run; see Chapter 6).

Realistically, Barb can see a time when her motivation will wane, especially if, through injury or aging, she could no longer be a top masters runner. Barb quickly added that she would not give up easily and would take two or three years to try to return to top form. She also noted that "being humbled is not a bad idea every now and then."

Personal Processes

Like all the other masters athletes featured in this book, Barb has very high personal standards. Her standards can be briefly described as always training as hard as possible (short of injuring herself) and trying during racing season to establish personal records in distances ranging from the 5K to the marathon. Barb's reference group is composed of the top masters runners in the world, although she adds that she is constantly striving to improve.

Her detailed log also provides an important vehicle for objectively observing her performances and progress. For example, she will frequently examine workouts that preceded certain races over the years and find some of the reasons for good or poor performances.

While Barb finds that "it's exciting and satisfying to set a new personal record at this older age . . . it shows you're not losing it yet," and she gets a terrifically happy glow from meeting or exceeding her standards, she does not get depressed about subpar performances. Instead, she examines her training log and makes some changes. Win or lose, Barb considers herself a good sport and respectful of her competitors.

At home, her latest trophy or ribbon gets prominent display. But after a few days, the excitement wears off, and she is back to hard training. Through trial and error, Barb has developed a training program that works for her, and she is very confident in both the program and her abilities.

Barb, her competitors, and readers may wonder how long she can improve and be a very top athlete. Barb seems to have the psychological and constitutional background to continue for many years to come:

> I think I am following my dad's attitude, his six brothers, and his late father. Their age range is 69 to 84. They're all spry, athletic, in good health, and refuse to grow old. They still golf, bowl, pitch horseshoes, and dance all night.

By all accounts, Barb may well have 15 years of improvement ahead of her!

JOSEPH GERMANA

Joseph Germana, Ph.D., represents an important and very exciting segment of ageless athletes. At the age of 47, Joe is a competitive bodybuilder and the faculty adviser for the Virginia Tech Weightlifting Club and the Virginia Tech Boxing Club. That does not sound very unusual until you know that until five years ago, Joe, at best, was involved only sporadically in some fitness activities such as cycling and jogging. Seven years ago he was a heavy smoker. Thus, *until* reaching middle age, Joe did not have any athletic interests. Today, a few short years later, he is one of the top masters bodybuilders in Virginia. Indeed, in recent contests, Joe was the most "ripped" (defined) and best poser of any entrant (ages 16–53) in the contests. Joe has found, as have many other middle-aged athletes, that it's never too late to become an athlete.

Joe was born in New York City in 1940 and received his Ph.D. in psychology from Rutgers University in 1965. His major areas of interest are in experimental psychology, psychophysiology, personality, and systems theory. Besides his research and writings in psychology, Joe is one of the most energetic and dynamic lecturers I have ever heard. He brings a matchless enthusiasm and intensity to his teaching. Over a period of 23 years, students have consistently rated Joe as one of the university's top instructors.

Joe has been married to Gail for 24 years and has two children, Stephanie, 23, and Michael, 17. Joe is kind of a "homebody," devoted to a tranquil life.

Joe is also multitalented. Aside from his work in psychology, he has written in such fields as art and philosophy, as well as satire and critical reviews. He is an artist who specializes in abstract painting, mainly in the acrylic media, and has had a number of showings of his work. He has recently become a sought-after model. These various pursuits, as we will shortly see, fit together for Joe in his ideal of a balanced and harmonious life.

Goals and Standards

Joe describes his athletic goals mainly as personal and spiritual. He believes that his full and authentic involvement in a physical discipline benefits him psychologically, socially, physically, and, therefore, spiritually. Competition is simply one more step toward fuller involvement.

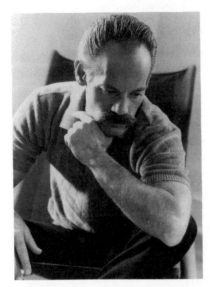

Joe in a contemplative mood.

Thus, Joe's personal standards are somewhat different from other masters athletes featured in this book. True, he always wants to do his best, but winning is not his major goal. Indeed, realistically assessing his potential, Joe feels he will probably never win a major masters competition.

Instead, as noted, "authentic involvement," the act and the doing, seem the most important sources of motivation for Joe. For example, Joe's posing routines are precisely choreographed works of art. He gets incredible pleasure from just performing these routines.

Effects of Aging and Training

With Joe and other individuals who are emerging as athletes in their middle years, it is difficult to assess the effects, if any, of aging. There is simply no baseline of previous performances. However, we do have Joe's report that he looks and feels stronger and more fit than at any previous point in his life. In addition to his increased physical activity, his improved diet may also contribute to that feeling. Since he was 40, Joe has followed a strict ovo-lacto-vegetarian diet. During the last few years, that diet has been modified a bit so that it now can be described as a high-complex carbohydrate, low-fat, moderate protein, but still meatless diet. His nutritional practices are, thus, far superior to what they were in his 20s and 30s.

Joe has been able to follow arduous bodybuilding routines that would defeat athletes half his age. For example, for about a year, Joe did a split (upper, lower body) routine every other day, with each workout sometimes lasting up to two hours. During this period, which Joe thought of as an experiment to see how well he responded to one approach, he never missed a workout. When a chronic lower back problem that Joe has had for over 25 years flares up, he simply switches his leg routine to more isolated exercises such as leg extensions and leg curls and drops, or uses light weights on squats and leg presses. Although when he gets appreciably older injuries may take their toll, Joe feels he will always train and do specialized workouts to keep going and compensate for injuries.

Joe's bodybuilding routine has always been supplemented by some aerobic work, such as cycling, jogging, and walking. Recently, his training and athletic pursuits have taken another unusual turn. In addition to bodybuilding, Joe has been taking boxing lessons, including sparring, rope jumping, and intervals with the heavy bag.

Perhaps what is so exciting about Joe and other masters athletes who do not have a long history of athletics is their sheer joy in being an athlete. This is often accompanied by a very fresh and open approach to experimentation with new routines or totally different approaches. Ironically, there are a number of benefits to starting later in life. Every new routine is, indeed, new. And without a backlog of records from their 20s and 30s, there are no real self-imposed limits. Anything may be possible! Joe is an example of overcoming "limits." He has always been very defined in contests, but too thin. During the last six months, however, Joe has been able to gain about one and a half pounds of muscle per month—very respectable gains at any age!

Other Sources of Motivation

Like a number of other masters athletes, Joe does *not* have

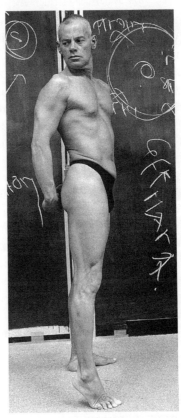

Though still thin, Joe has
been gaining a pound of
muscle a month.

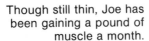

problems motivating himself for a hard workout. Because Joe's
children are older and he has a flexible work schedule, Joe can
usually schedule workouts at fairly optimal times. Once a
workout starts, Joe moves from exercise to exercise rather
quickly. The setting, experience, and moment-to-moment
feedback seem to generate his motivation. Joe describes it as a
sort of "functional autonomy." He said, "Whether I am looking forward to a particular workout or not, whether I have to
work around an injury or not, once I begin to warm up and
stretch, and start lifting weights, one thing leads to another."
Psychologists call this *stimulus control*. That is, situational cues
tend to evoke certain habitual responses that have often occurred in a particular setting. Thus, one simple approach for
overcoming a lack of motivation is to just put yourself in the
situation and start.

Joe, however, does point to other sources of motivation. As a faculty advisor to the Weightlifting Club, which is the largest club on campus with about 1,500 members, part of Joe's responsibilities is to function as a role model to members. This includes his appearance, his approach to training, the advice he gives to members, and generally how he conducts himself in and out of the gym. A few select friends also share his interest and are sources of information, encouragement, and feedback.

Joe says that he receives more attention and feedback from people younger than he is. Some people of the same age appear a bit perplexed with Joe's bodybuilding and, particularly now, his competitions. Joe feels these people do not understand the degree of motivation and commitment needed in the "Iron Game," or the satisfaction that participation can provide.

Joe indicated that he responds well to more positive feedback. He is aware that he will try to influence the feedback process by working harder and looking better. In boxing, this feedback process is much more physically intense and personal. Joe works out with a small group of boxers (the newly formed Virginia Tech Boxing Club) who are devoted to the sport. Sparring with the coach provides instantaneous positive reinforcement and, of course, punishment. Thus, much of the feedback and reinforcement Joe receives is interpersonal. His feedback is also personal in that he fulfills certain standards and role expectations for himself. Media exposure, public commitments, or relying on a training diary for feedback are not Joe's sources of feedback and reinforcement.

Like many other masters athletes, Joe has reached a point in his life where training conditions are ideal. His flexible work schedule and older children allow him the freedom to train at optimal times. In addition, he always has access to the bodybuilding facilities at Virginia Tech, which are among the best in the country and resemble a well-equipped Gold's gym. Joe readily admits that at least part of the success he has achieved as a masters athlete is attributable to his ability "to control the environment."

Joe also has a general role model that he emulates, the Japanese writer-athlete-spiritual leader, Yukio Mishima (1925–1970). This role model is best described in Eastern terms as the "superior person," who has integrated various arts and skills, is capable of taking action, and who has achieved harmony and balance in his life. As a friend and observer, it has been fascinating to see Joe continually evolve and approach his role model.

Joe at 47.

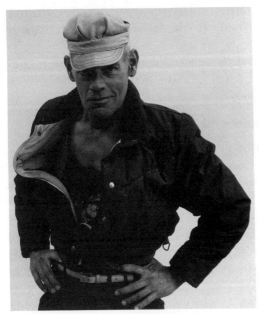

JOHN M. GREGG

I was sitting out on my front lawn one day when I first saw an amazing-looking figure charging up the steep hill adjacent to my house. I thought for sure that Arnold Schwarzenegger was finally going to pay me a visit. I had simply never before seen such a large and muscular person running any distance. I quickly recognized a friend of mine rather desperately trying to keep up with this formidable fellow. My sympathy went out to the friend, and I knew I had to find out more about this middle-aged superman.

Dr. John M. Gregg was born in Schenectady, New York, in May 1940. He has a B.A. degree from the University of Michigan, as well as a D.D.S., an M.S. in anatomy, another M.S. in oral surgery, and a Ph.D. in anatomy-neuroanatomy, all from the same university. John is currently a practicing oral and maxillofacial surgeon in Blacksburg, Virginia. In the past, he has practiced in Ann Arbor, Michigan, and Chapel Hill, North Carolina, and has had full-time appointments at the University of Michigan and the University of North Carolina. John is well-known nationally for his research in microsurgery nerve repair.

John is now separated from his wife. He is the father of two children—Edward, 22, and Kristin, 19.

Athletic Career and Training Philosophy

John's athletic career spans a period of over 30 years. His first pursuits, not surprisingly, were sprints and football. John was an All-American in high school at 100 and 200 meters and the New York State champion and 200-yard record holder in 1957. In college, John was twice the Big 10 silver medalist in the sixty-yard dash, and was also twice on the sprint relay Big 10 championship team. John was ranked tenth nationally in the decathalon in 1963, was the 100-meter record holder for the 1970 Southeast region masters track and field games, and most recently, took second place in the National (Masters) Championship Track Pentathlon (1985).

Through the years, John's best marks have been 9.4 for 100 yards, 10.4 for 100 meters, 20.8 for 200 meters, 47.7 for 400 meters, 17:06 for the 5K, 37:00 for the 10K, and a 3:06:00 marathon. Recently, John has branched out into bike racing, triathlons, and some weight training (I think he would be incredible if he seriously stayed with the weights for a year), and hiking and backpacking as recreational pursuits. Thus, John has trained hard for many years.

John's training goals, approach, and overall philosophy are quite different from most of the masters athletes featured in this book. At 6'1" and a muscular 190 pounds, it is obvious that

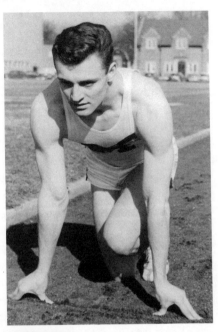

John in high school.

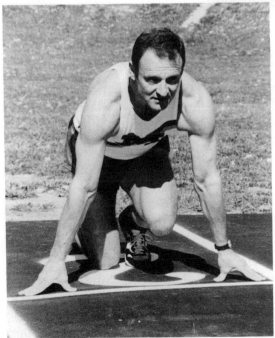

John thirty years later.

he would do best in strength and more anaerobic activities. However, very early on, John decided *not* to channel himself just into his "one best activity."

Instead, for the past 25 years he has tried to approach an ideal of a *total* level of fitness, including speed, strength, flexibility, and endurance. He works to develop a base from which on short notice and with very little specialized training he could, for example, run a top 100-meter dash or do well in a long bike race. He thrives on diversity, but said that to take his approach, athletes must swallow some pride and be willing to train and compete in some events where they are only average. For John, this is fine. He feels as much satisfaction from doing his best at running a reasonable 5K time as he does in winning a 200-meter dash.

The reason may be the philosophical perspective one of John's teachers gave him at an early age. It can be called the "90 percent rule." That is, a person with a reasonable degree of talent and ability and a willingness to work hard can get to be about 90 percent of the very best in a wide range of areas in life. However, to get to the 100 percent level in one area will most often require incredible effort that usually will preclude much participation in other areas. John has preferred to be 90 percent in a number of areas, "to sample different lines of life." Although through natural talent John is probably at a 95 percent level in sprinting, by generally keeping to his 90 percent rule in athletics, he has also developed an outstanding medical career, continued to play trumpet in a band, and raised two children.

Training and Aging

Because of John's exceptional and varied background, degree of intensity, and string of accomplishments, he is in a better position than most of us to evaluate any effects of aging. John noted three major effects: loss of speed, a longer time for skeletal-muscular recovery, and recurring achilles tendonitis. He has tried to compensate for these apparent effects of aging by adding some strength work to his schedule; maintaining his interval or cross-country hill fartlek workouts, but limiting them to twice a week, 40–50 minutes per session; and alternating activities, such as sprinting, biking, weight training, and easier running in his schedule. Overall, because of some strength training, John feels that he is quite a bit stronger than 15 years ago, but he has noted a decline in his aerobic strength during the last 10 years and a rather steady decline in his sprint speed during the last 20 years. He feels most of his "decline" started in his late 30s, but that a good part of that decline was attributable to personal and marital problems. During this last year, by contrast, John has met a woman who is interested in athletics and his training and performances have taken off again!

Like all the masters athletes featured in this book, John has psychologically compensated for any physical decline by heightened discipline and motivation. He mentally visualizes a hard workout the day before. During intense sessions, he most often trains with partners, stays a bit hungry that day, and has a strong cup of coffee two or three hours before the workout. He sets specific goals two or three months before a competition, has longer range general goals that are geared toward a total aerobic/anaerobic strength conditioning and performance, and keeps himself interested and motivated by changing his type of training and competition every two to three years (e.g., from sprinting to 10 miles to triathlons).

John further explained that about every two or three years he comes off his total conditioning base and trains more specifically for certain events. Typically, this has meant training for sprints. John noted that he can quickly become competitive in his age group, but when really trying to excel, he often gets injured. John realizes that to reach the top in specific events he needs a more focused program. However, that would violate his 90 percent rule.

More typically, at any one time, he competes in such varied events as 100- and 200-meter dashes, triathlons, and bike races. John may go on a long bike tour for recreation.

Although, as noted, John does do some very intense workouts, his schedule remains varied and flexible. Almost every day he does something, but he notes "I never have a rigid game plan." He is both attracted and driven to training as an escape, a release, and for the satisfaction and euphoria that accompany good workouts.

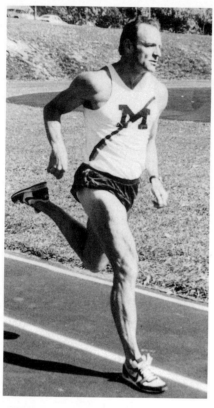

John gets a great feeling of exhilaration from a good interval session.

Other Motivation Factors

Those particular emotional experiences also keep John training at a high level. He loves the euphoria that immediately accompanies hard workouts and the lingering heightened feelings following the workout. John likes the rewards of being very fit, being able, for example, to backpack, ski, and maintain his youthful appearance. He has also found that when he does not train, he feels depressed. Other sources of motivation include his occasional training partners, periodic participation as a team member in track clubs, a variety of sports-related books and magazines, and public commitments such as announcing his race plans to friends and family. Unlike a number of masters athletes, John does not keep a detailed training log or diary.

Sources of feedback and reinforcement for John are clearly interpersonal. Reinforcement and feedback come from the companionship and approval of his son, training partners, and professional colleagues. John feels a special pride in being able to balance his professional and athletic life-style. John has not been featured in local or national media, and has not received any monetary compensations. He also cannot point to any particular role models. Thus, his immediate friends and family, his good feelings and accomplishments from training, and his high and unique personal standards are what keep John motivated.

Although John's children are older, his hectic work schedule makes his training routine less than ideal. John would prefer training in the early afternoon, but currently most of his training occurs in the evening. However, as you probably guessed, he is tenacious. He will work at night, if necessary, to get in his evening workout. Surgery, emergency calls, and other work commitments prohibit a completely fixed training routine.

Sample Training Program

Despite these limitations imposed by the demands of his work, John's training schedule remains very ambitious. A typical week's schedule includes anaerobic training of twice per week intervals of moderate effort (70 percent) on the track, a mix of 200, 300, and 400 meters for 10 repetitions. John's aerobic training usually includes one long (7–12 miles) run per week, and five- to six-mile runs alternated with one-hour bike rides, two to three times per week. His training runs are interspersed with fartleks or hill running. John's strength training is mostly confined to upper body work twice per week in the summer and more weight training in the winter. This is a very balanced and varied schedule and allows John to meet his standards of being prepared for a variety of emphases and competitions.

Medical Career and Practice

Not surprisingly, John left his prestigious academic position at the height of his career to get back to pursuing his foremost interests. John felt that he was a prime example of the "Peter Principle." Because he was successful in academia, he was doing more and more administrative work, and less and less hands-on treatment and research. He realized that he most enjoyed working directly with patients and the science and art of surgery.

John's current practice is thriving. He has, however, kept active in research and continues data collection and basic studies through his practice. In a sense, part of his practice has become an important research foundation, and he is still on the leading edge of microsurgery nerve repair research. John has also had several attractive offers to return to universities. It will be interesting to see how his varied career interests and abilities play out over the next several years.

Parting Words

As is the case for almost all the masters athletes in this book, training for John is a lifetime pursuit. He said he simply couldn't foresee circumstances that would significantly decrease his motivation for training.

John left me with some parting words that should be helpful to many masters athletes: "Train hard, but not too hard. And play your flute and drink a glass of wine also."

LUCILLE GRIFFIN

Lucille Griffin was born in August 1938, in Glen Cove, New York. She has been married to Gary since August 1959. Lucille has a bachelors degree from Colorado State University, where she majored in French. She also attended the Sorbonne for a year. Lucille is the mother of four grownup children—Lise, Victoria, Heather, and Glenn—and has recently retired from active swim coaching.

Lucille's story is an amazing one. Although she's been a competitive swimmer for 35 years, she is still improving and setting PRs at 50 years of age. But wait, there's more. This lady has won national championships *after* being out of training for over a year with serious and chronic injuries. These injuries are still with her and, perhaps, always will be. However, when Lucille's injuries abate, she is capable of outstanding performances. This is because she has developed a unique training program that helps compensate for her injuries and prevents serious injury. She is a great advertisement for her book, *Teach Yourself to Swim the Racing Strokes* (Gap Mountain Books).

And, indeed, although Lucille had expert and inspired coaching when she started, for the last 20 years she has taught herself new strokes and better form. Thus, she really believes strongly in the ability of others to improve their swimming by developing strokes and turns.

Lucille's most striking accomplishments occurred in the Short Course (25-yard pool) Nationals Swim meet held in Fort Pierce, Florida, in May 1986. She entered six events in the 45–49 age group, winning three of the events, and finishing second, third, and fifth in the others. Lucille won the 50-yard backstroke, the 100-yard backstroke, and the 200-yard butterfly. Her time in the 200-yard butterfly was *seven* seconds faster than her previous PR! In three other events, the 50-yard and 100-yard butterfly and the 50-yard backstroke, she also established PRs. Finally, she was within a half-second of her time in the 100-yard backstroke that had given her All-America honors five years previously. For the 1986 Top Ten Masters short course swimmers ratings, she was in the top five for five separate events! For the 1986 long course *World* Masters ratings, she was in the top five for six events and tenth in another!

These marks were accomplished despite ligament damage in her right elbow, scar tissue in both elbows, and two partially degenerated discs in her neck which cause the vertebra between them to go out of alignment. Then how does she do it? How does she train, and what keeps her motivated?

Training

One principle that Lucille has found that many other masters have embraced is that *less* is often *best*, if the quality is there.

During the summer, she tries to swim daily, but her maximum is only 45 minutes or 1,500 meters. During the winter, Lucille is in the pool four or five times per week for a maximum of 45 minutes or 2,000 yards. She has dropped her interval and repeat training and confines her speed work to kicking and some very limited fast strokes at the end of a length (25 yards or less). Lucille always concentrates on maintaining excellent form and constantly strives to improve it. Her training in these sessions is precise. She always counts strokes per length of the pool and monitors intensity by taking her pulse.

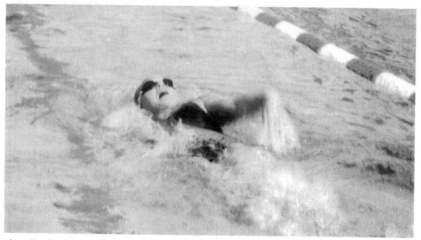

Lucille in the backstroke at a national championship.

Only about 25 percent of Lucille's workload can be considered high-intensity. Most of her conditioning is achieved through the butterfly stroke, which Lucille feels is hard work but easier on her injuries. Lucille is also very careful about practicing race starts. Swimming is a sport that not only requires great strength and endurance, but also meticulous attention to form. In describing a training session, she noted that:

> I am always trying to make the most out of my efforts. Everything aims at *feeling*. Whenever it feels just right, it always looks great, and this is the only way I am able to achieve any speed. In

practice, therefore, slow or fast, I am concentrating on the feeling. Obviously, right away, weakness or lack of conditioning is felt. Pulse monitoring provides a double check.

In addition to her swim training, Lucille is doing circuit weight training two days per week. This consists of using a wide variety of exercises while being careful to train around her injuries—generally using light weights with high repetitions. After returning to training, Lucille could barely move some of the machines even without resistance. Eventually, she could bench press, curl, and military press with medium resistance. Currently, she is also experimenting with cycling to increase endurance and strength in her legs.

Perhaps if three words can describe Lucille's current program, those words are *intelligent, focused,* and *consistent.* Like most masters athletes described in this book, she rarely misses a workout.

This workout plan is quite a bit different from the one Lucille used only a few years ago. Then she swam every day in the summer up to 2,200 meters of which 1,500 (70 percent) was high intensity such as intervals, repeats, breath control, or distance swims at 90 percent effort. Her summer program was supplemented by cycling. Her winter program involved swimming up to 2,500 yards, much of it also high-intensity work, four or five times per week, with some limited weight training included. So, Lucille has not only been able to continue by doing less, she's actually improved.

Motivation: External Factors

As with other athletes featured in this book, and as discussed at length in Chapter 2, we know that questions about motivation are not simple; they require looking at the intersection of external factors and internal personal processes. I will start here with external factors.

It is clear that Lucille has benefitted from brief, careful, and intelligently planned swim workouts, supplemented with weight training. She's found a system to keep her injuries at a manageable level and has stuck with it. She also follows a regular calisthenic program upon waking and before going to bed. Lucille feels this routine stimulates circulation and reduces stiffness. She now also includes a 10-minute stretching routine and a minimum warm up of swimming 500 yards prior to any workouts and competition. She does not train for two to three days after any major meet. Thus, quite obviously, a successful tailor-made program fuels motivation—outcome expectancies and efficacy beliefs.

Because Lucille is self-employed and her children are grown, she can schedule her workouts at fairly optimal times and fit the rest of her schedule around her workouts. She also has ready access to a pool at Virginia Tech and a weight system at the town's recreation center. Compared to years ago, when her access to facilities was tenuous and family responsibilities dominated the day, her training schedule and conditions are close to ideal. As we have seen in this book, this is one advantage many masters athletes seem to have. They have better control over their training environment and circumstances, most often because of the period of life they are in.

Because Lucille's workouts are very well planned and manageable, she does not need to be "up" to have a good workout. She always looks forward to them and almost always has a good workout. This is another instance where reachable goals yield success, and success breeds more success. In addition, Lucille, like many masters athletes, always feels mentally and physically better after a workout. Lucille said that this great feeling provides ample reason to get into a workout and keep training. Each part of her program provides an important ingredient for her fitness and well-being.

Lucille noted that all her best friends are swimmers, although most often she trains alone. This means, however, that going to meets becomes a great social occasion. She also frankly admits that she constantly tries to look good swimming in training or at meets as a way to promote her book by engaging the interest of other people.

Lucille has considerable support from her husband, who goes to most of her meets; her daughters and son, whose feedback and comments keep her on her toes; and her coach at meets, who is rich with praise and helpful pointers. Her Virginia Masters teammates provide friendship, encouragement, and a good time. Lucille naturally reciprocates such positive feedback.

Lucille also keeps up on most of the current literature on swimming techniques and masters events. She shares this information with friends and teammates in various articles she writes. The listing of results in masters meets provides good comparison points for her.

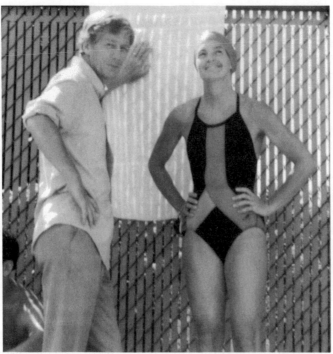

Relaxing between events with husband Gary.

Maintaining her current workout schedule and not becoming injured have become Lucille's major goals. Despite her meticulous workouts, she no longer keeps a detailed training log. Lucille feels that she does not need one because she tries to always do the best possible workout she can do under prevailing circumstances.

Lucille feels that considering her age and injuries, her abilities have declined. But as she notes:

> My muscles are stronger and better balanced and I can swim faster than ever. So I have declined and improved at the same time. The natural decline of aging has not yet cancelled the benefits of long experience and "knowing my body."

Lucille's sources of reinforcement identified before are mostly self-generated feedback and social reinforcement. Lucille maintains social reinforcement by providing it in turn to others. However, outside of her network, this national champion and world-class athlete is little known and hardly receives accolades even in her hometown. Articles about Lucille in the local newspapers have only appeared because of her own initiative. In contrast, the reactions of middle-aged and same-aged swimmers have been positive. Lucille hopes that some of the younger swimmers are inspired by her example, and this also serves to keep her motivated.

Lucille's father has been a long-time inspiration for her. She trains harder and tries harder at national meets by keeping him in mind. As a youngster, it was Lucille's father who got her started in athletics, gave Lucille her love of swimming, and introduced her to her first coach. Her father has remained Lucille's strongest supporter and has encouraged and backed her coaching and writing career.

Lucille has also had a lifelong role model who she has admired since childhood. This person is the former Olympic swimmer from Australia, Dawn Fraser. Lucille did not attempt to copy Dawn because Dawn was a freestyle sprinter, but she saw Dawn as an inspiration. Lucille may soon have an opportunity to swim with Dawn, who has recently entered masters competition. This should help to keep Lucille in top shape.

Internal Processes

Lucille is a very precise observer of her responses during workouts and uses these observations to fine-tune her workouts. Despite a relatively relaxed approach to training and competition and her history of injuries, Lucille still has very high personal standards for herself as a swimmer. Her standards, specific goals, and careful workouts leave her with "irrepressible great expectations" for her competitions. But there is something more important to Lucille in competition:

> I like to be in good shape, and I especially love to swim. I always look forward to competitions because they are a measurement of, and great incentive for, continued fitness. I also look on each competition as a learning experience—learning more about myself. Improvement can only come this way.

Lucille, not surprisingly, tries to keep her successes and failures in swimming in perspective. Very good workouts or competitions, she feels, often "are a gift of that particular day, and the favorable coincidence of many influences, including chance." Thus, Lucille tries to enjoy the triumphs and learn from the failures; she does not specifically reward or punish herself for performances. However, it must be noted that her relatively "mellow" approach is offset by considerable emotion at other times, as when, for example, injury and inactivity lead to depression.

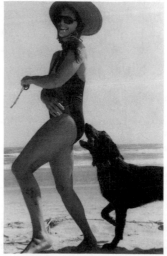

After a meet—barely staying out of reach of the family dog.

When Lucille is not injured, she is extremely confident in her overall approach and her own abilities. She has a good sense of what exercises help her for different strokes and how she needs to race for different events. For example, by reviewing recent races, Lucille found that she could only swim her best times in the 200-yard butterfly when her form is nearly perfect and when she actually makes herself *not* race the event. Considering that Lucille is ranked second nationally in this event, there appears to be an interesting lesson here for other athletes.

Lucille also readily admits that part of her extreme confidence in her abilities comes from genetics. Her natural flexibility, height (5'8"), great reach, large hands and large pigeon-toed feet give her almost an ideal swimmer's body. Yes, like most champions, part of the explanation for Lucille's success is that she was born that way.

But, as with other masters athletes featured in this book, Lucille has great perseverance and determination—perhaps more so, given her history of injuries and returns to top competition. She has always believed that her hard work would be rewarded sooner or later. She has always taken a long-term perspective which can be invaluable to athletes, particularly those disappointed with their first competitive ventures or with injuries. For example, despite superior genetics and a belief in her abilities, when Lucille returned to competitive swimming in her mid-30s, she still felt that to reach the top:

> It was a question of staying in shape and competition long enough. Originally, I. figured it might take 20 or 30 years to make my way to the top of the rankings, and this was a source of inspiration rather than discouragement.

Postscript

In 1987, Lucille was coming back from another set of injuries. It appears that once again she will emerge triumphant. However, the repetitive injuries have made her realistically foresee a time when her expectations will be decreased and she will no longer swim hard workouts. Her training may at some point be limited to lap swimming. But like so many other masters athletes, Lucille said, "I will always train."

And Lucille added an important point and perspective for other ageless athletes:

> I will always compete. I like to win as much as the next person, but it definitely is not everything. It is more important to keep swimming. Certainly, I won't quit just because others pass me. That wouldn't be fair to the rest.

JOHN F. HOSNER

John F. Hosner, Ph.D., is older than all but one of the other masters athletes featured in this book. However, just as the record of accomplishment of athletes in their 40s and 50s can serve as an inspiration to younger athletes, John's accomplishments in his 60s should provide the younger masters athletes with an exemplar motivational role model. John is not only setting age group records, he is also still setting PRs!

John F. Hosner was born in Gillespie, Illinois, in February 1925. He received his B.S. degree in Forestry from Michigan State University in 1948, his M.S. degree in Forest Soils from Duke University in 1950, and his Ph.D. in Forest Ecology from the State University of New York at Syracuse in 1957. Presently, John is Associate Dean of the College of Agriculture and Life Sciences and Director of the School of Forestry and Wildlife Resources at Virginia Tech. Prior to coming to Virginia Tech, John held a number of field and academic positions from 1948 to 1961.

John has two grown children, David, 34, and Angela, 36, from his first marriage. He was remarried in 1978 to Katrina.

John has had an interesting, varied, and successful sports background, although he never really hit his stride until becoming a serious runner. In high school, John participated in football as a running back and in track in the half-mile and mile. John said he distinguished himself in neither activity. He explained that his physical development was quite slow; he

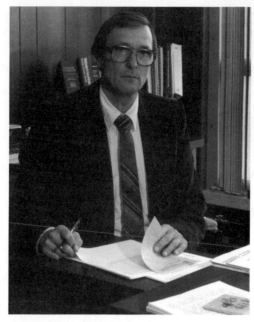

John "as a dean." John has helped make the Forestry and Wildlife Resources School at Virginia Tech one of the best in the country.

was a year younger than most of his classmates, and upon graduation weighed 127 pounds.

While in college, John tried his hand in a wide range of sandlot and intramural sports. He particularly enjoyed the competition and discovered some talent for boxing. In 1947, John was the intramural champion at Michigan State University in the 145-pound class.

After college, John continued in competitive sports. In softball and racquetball, he frequently played in tournaments and won many district and regional competitions. John has maintained his interest in tournament-level softball but last year decided to retire from that sport, both to avoid injury and to devote himself more to running.

Competition

John quite frankly admits that he thrives on competition and feels that sports competition helps him in other parts of his life. John said that:

> I enjoy all types of sports competition. I feel the competition carries over into my job. Our programs in forestry and wildlife at Virginia Tech are rated by our peers as being in the top five in the U.S. That gives me a great feeling of pride and a desire to be the best.

Since John had succeeded in a range of athletic pursuits, I was curious as to why he decided to concentrate on running about 10 years ago. John's explanation also revolved around competition:

> I liked the number of opportunities for competition in running. In racquetball, there were much fewer opportunities. Also, in both racquetball and softball, I was usually competing with 25-year-olds, and to be quite honest, I wasn't competitive anymore. The age division racing and the numerous races that were available were the main factors in my switch to running. I also quickly found out that I was really a top runner in my age group, and I like to win.

Records

John is more than a "top" age group runner. On March 5, 1985, on the indoor track at VMI (Virginia Military Institute) in Lexington, Virginia, John set a world record for the 60–64 age group class. He covered 1,500 meters in 5:05! He holds a string of age and state records across a wide range of distances. John's best times are 17:19 for 5,000 meters (with a PR of 16:59 when 59 years old); 28:46 for 8,000 meters; 35:09 for 10,000 meters; 58:55 for 10 miles; and 1:18:10 for a half-marathon.

The diversity of these records is clearly astounding. But wait, there's more. The 10K and 10-mile times were actually PRs. That's right. At age 60, John was still cranking out PRs after almost 35 years of athletics and about 10 years of competitive running. The National Running Data Center rated John as the nation's top male road runner, 60–64, for 1985.

John's records would be the envy of any world class professional athlete. However, John has accomplished his records despite his hectic professional life, which often involves up to 50 hours of work per week and a fair amount of travel!

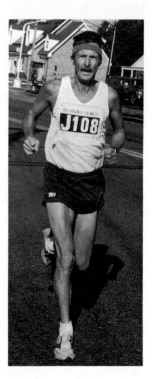

Cruising along at a great pace in the annual Virginia ten-miler at Lynchburg.

Like most masters athletes, John no longer has the pressures of having a young family. But his work schedule makes training circumstances far from ideal. Fitting in his workout is a major priority each day.

Training

John's training is mostly confined to the noon hour during the week. For a runner at his level, his training, particularly the pace (see below), is quite conservative. John's workouts seem low-key and enjoyable rather than grueling. Perhaps we find in this kind of approach one important key for the longevity and continued motivation of some athletes: keep it short, simple, and most importantly, *enjoyable*. Thus, it appears that a good deal of John's speed work comes from his competitive races, although he has recently added higher intensity intervals and sporadic fartlek training to his program.

When training for racing, a typical week's schedule for John involves:

Sunday:	long run at 8-minute pace for 12–15 miles.
Monday:	easy run at 8-minute pace for 5–7 miles.
Tuesday:	Intervals 4 × 440 at 1:20, 2 × 880 at 2:50, 1 mile at 5:40–6:00, Plus 1-mile warm-up and cool-down and jogging the repetition distance as the interval.
Wednesday:	easy run at 8-minute pace for 7–8 miles.
Thursday:	moderate run at about 7:30 pace for 7–8 miles.
Friday:	moderate run at 7:30–8-minute pace for 10 miles.
Saturday:	easy run at 8-minute pace for 7 miles.

Interestingly, when training with other area runners, John sometimes has trouble keeping up with them. In competition, John often *beats* them. This observation suggests how on the one hand John has found a training program that is sufficient to keep him very fit and relatively injury-free. On the other hand, the same observation suggests a great ability to focus, become highly motivated, and extract the best from himself in competition.

Concentration

John explained his incredible performance capabilities by saying that first:

> I like to know the course, then I mentally run the course numerous times in preparation for the race. I also plan mentally how I will respond to possible competition. . . . I am usually completely relaxed before a race to the point that I'm so sluggish I wonder if I'll even be able to run. However, when I start my warm-ups, I start "getting into it" and by the time the gun goes off, I'm ready to go.

John further explained that:

> I seldom concentrate on times. I concentrate on bettering my
> competition. My good times come as a result of being pushed
> by competition. However, very often I "select" as competition
> people 20–30 years younger. I not only try to keep up with
> them, but beat them!

Other Sources of Motivation

Although John noted that he does not focus on his race times,
he sets a reachable goal of winning his age group whenever he
competes in a masters competition. It is also possible that he
can set a personal or age group record. Such goal attainments
are clearly motivational.

Perhaps another facet of training and competition that has
kept John highly motivated is that he keeps his racing seasonal. He employs a period of "active rest" every year when
he runs slowly and does not track time or distance. (See Chapter 3 on periodization.) Thus, John only fully extends himself
during certain parts of the year and remains physically and
psychologically fresh.

John's wife Katrina is also an occasional training partner and
has encouraged him to go to big national-level competitions.
She also accompanies him to these races, sometimes doing the
driving. Katrina is also quite competitive and can usually win
or place in her age division.

John maintains a training log where he records the distance,
intensity, and speed of his training runs. He also records his
race results, overall place, age division results, and his splits
and times. John reviews his past training and competition records during his build-up for a racing season and will try to
match and then surpass these records.

Because John is so competitive, he sometimes uses a public
commitment strategy to prime himself for a race. For example,
he will tell friends that he intends to win his age group in a
particular race—which, of course, often occurs.

John receives a considerable amount of positive feedback

(praise, compliments) from his wife, friends, and his brothers. John has always been very competitive with his older brother, Joseph, and his younger brother, Albert. Both his brothers are very athletic, and, indeed, Albert has been a three-time national senior paddleball champion. Albert now is starting to become more involved in running, so their personal competition may be more strongly renewed. Feedback and praise from his brothers is particularly motivational for John.

John also makes it a point to talk to people who understand and appreciate his records. Area runners really understand what running a 35-minute 10K at age 62 means. Seeking out such fellow athletes is one way that John influences the feedback process. John also admits that he enjoys laudatory newspaper and magazine writeups of his accomplishments and finds them motivating.

As with other masters athletes, general feedback from other people is mixed. The reactions of many younger people to John's training and accomplishments are positive and admiring. Some peers are also quite positive while "others think I'm crazy." John feels that the positive reactions from younger people and other masters runners are clearly motivational; the negative reactions from nonrunners do not bother him.

Personal Processes

While systematic training and environmental supports are clearly important ingredients in any athlete's success, personal beliefs and standards may be at the core of athletic motivation. This is, of course, particularly the case when beliefs and standards can be supported by the environment and behavioral outcomes as we discussed in Chapter 2.

During preparatory training for races, John is an astute observer of his training and recovery. For training, the key dimension that he tracks is speed.

John is the first to admit that he is incredibly competitive. He always has one goal for himself—to win! He has always been very competitive in his work and other sports, and this approach just naturally carried over to his running. However, his competitiveness in running has taken on almost a life of its own. That's because when John started, he did not realize how good he would become. He competed locally, then on state and national levels. Now he wants to compete internationally. He first broke state records, then national records, and now is after another world record. His success has fueled his competitiveness and his own personal standards keep going up and up (an example of the "upward spiralling" effect discussed in Chapter 2).

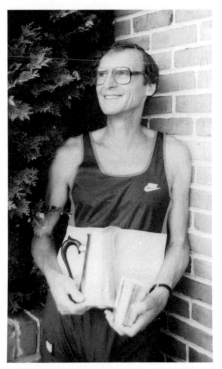

After all his wins, John still relishes winning a big race.

As with many other masters athletes to whom performance is very important, John acknowledges that his mood and affect are very much related to meeting or exceeding his standards, or failing to do so. But his irritability and depression following suboptimal performances do not last long. John rewards himself with food or drink for great performances but doesn't punish himself for subpar competitions.

John has a great deal of confidence in his present program, as it is the one that made him the nation's top runner in his age division. Except when injured, John has never doubted that he would be successful. On the one hand, John assigns much of the basis for his success to genetic superiority, for example, a very high VO$_2$ max. On the other hand, John noted that because training and racing are still secondary in his life, he has no idea now well he actually could run if training and racing were his number one priority.

Aging and Training

How has John managed to keep improving, and are there any obvious signs of aging that John is experiencing, dealing with, and compensating for? As for training, as discussed, John's program is surely adequate, ambitious for "someone his age," clearly enjoyable, but not the total focus of his life. John is very competitive and is highly motivated and goal-directed; he points his efforts to particular races and records. Adding more speed work appears to have compensated for a loss of speed as John became older. When he achieved his various records, his training was very systematic. Of course, this suggests that John may have run somewhat faster when he was younger if he had emphasized speed work and more systematic training during that part of his career.

John also is more nutritionally conscious than he was 10 years ago. Like most of today's athletes, he basically follows a low-fat, high-complex carbohydrate diet. Without being fanatical, John tries to limit his simple sugars, salt, and red meat. These dietary practices are in some contrast to his younger years when John ate more fatty foods.

John has also recently noticed more stiffness and less flexibility. Not surprisingly, he has increased his stretching exercises, which basically involve stretching major muscle groups, with an emphasis on his hamstrings. This program helps to keep a chronic hamstring problem under control. John also does sit-ups and push-ups and 10–15 minutes of stretching after running.

The Future

However, a larger question—the main focus of this book—involves John's motivation to continue to train and compete at a very high level. It has to honestly be concluded that the question remains an open one. John indicated that he does see some of his motivation decreasing. He said:

> You have to realize that in about 12 years of (competitive) running, I've only finished second in an age group eight times, and third but once. I won all the other races, some with nine-year handicaps. One more trophy or win just doesn't seem that important anymore.

Well, before readers say, "I guess it has to happen sometime," and his competitors give a sigh of relief, John quickly noted, "I can still get up for the really big ones!"

AL OERTER

Al Oerter is the athlete featured in this book who is probably most associated with the term *ageless athlete*. Many readers will recall that Al achieved an unprecedented four Olympic gold medals in the discus in the 1956 Melbourne Olympics, the 1960 Rome games, 1964 in Tokyo, and again in the 1968 Olympics in Mexico City. In the 1968 games, when Al was 32, I recall broadcasters marveling that Al was able to compete "at his age." Then came an eight-year hiatus from all sports and a return to training and competition at the age of 40.

The United States did not participate in the 1980 Olympics, but Al won an alternate place on the U.S. team by placing fourth in the Olympic Trials. In 1984, just as Al was reaching his top shape, he suffered a leg injury that kept him out of contention for the Los Angeles games. Today, at 51, Al is starting to slowly peak for the 1988 Olympics.

It must be emphasized that Al is not training to compete in a "Masters Olympics," but for open competition against athletes 20 to 30 years younger than himself.

Of course, Al is often asked how and why he continues to compete. As we will see, the answers to these questions are really quite simple.

Training and Nutrition

The "how" part for all the masters athletes featured in this book is, on the surface, easily explained. Every older athlete, perhaps Al in particular, feels that their training is much "smarter" and finer tuned compared to their training when they were younger. And for those masters athletes still competing, often their "work ethic" is now superior to what it was in their youthful days.

With Al, the evidence for his superior training and nutrition program is immediately apparent. Over 20 years ago, Al was extremely bulky and strong, but not really looking sharp or in very good overall condition. What a difference in appearance now! Al looks very muscular, is in great condition, and in practice throws seems as agile and quick as the proverbial cat. Rather than manifesting the "inevitable physical declines with age," Al looks much improved and in some ways more "youthful."

Part of the credit for this transformation must go to improved nutrition. For a good part of Al's life, he was a typical "meat and potatoes guy." He grew up on "German family fare" meals and the notion that more was almost always better.

For many years, Al attributed not always feeling well and being tense to pressures at work, extended meetings, and the rigors of training. Today, he believes that most of those feelings can be explained by poor nutritional practices and drinking five to six cups of coffee per day. He now realizes that all that caffeine had him on a physical, and at times emotional, roller coaster.

Presently, Al's diet consists mostly of fish, poultry, whole grains, fresh fruits and vegetables, and supplements, the latter being a dietary practice that he has continued since his earlier days. His supplements include a judicious combination of vitamins, minerals, protein with a good amino acid combination, brewers yeast, dissected liver, and rose hips. His supplements are tuned to the demands of weather, training intensity, and other factors. He now has completely stopped drinking coffee.

Al's training includes heavy lifting, throwing, and some aerobics. Al has found a schedule over the years that he thrives on and enjoys. Clearly, as has been noted throughout this book, the "enjoy" part is a key to athletic longevity. He limits his training to about an hour and a half a day, a time that is very manageable, but only a fraction of the time spent training by many of his competitors.

Al simply alternates lifting and throwing days, seven days a week. His weight training focuses on basic, compound movements—squats, leg curls, bench presses or incline presses, flys, cable rows, lat machine pulldowns, upright rows, and curls. He stays away from heavy pulls and deadlifts to protect his shoulder area. He has, however, incorporated more Eagle Equipment (stackable weight machines) into his training because Al feels that they improve his flexibility while providing less joint stress.

Al pointed out that if he really pushed on weight training he may be able to go as high as close to 700 pounds in the squat and 500 in the bench. While it is rewarding to push big weights, and Al reports that he is stronger than ever before, Al emphasized that he is not a power lifter. His major focus is throwing, and power weight training just assists his throwing.

Al has a sophisticated approach to weight training: he uses a kind of periodization approach (see Chapter 3). A year or longer can be divided into preparation, throwing, and competitive phases. During the preparation phase, Al's goal is to become as strong as possible, so he uses very heavy weights and very quick movements. As Al starts concentrating more on throwing, he cuts back on the weights he uses. In the competitive season, he may cut back weights by as much as 50 percent.

Al feels that he is a much better thrower today than during

his younger days. He describes his youthful approach as depending on "brute force." He did not know a lot then about technique, much less practice technique. In recent years, Al has gone through a series of computerized biomechanical tests to find his optimal form. His practice sessions are likely to focus on getting into his optimal biomechanical groove and working on weak points in his form.

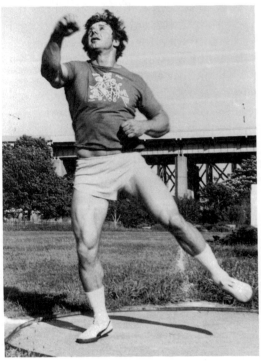

Al's throwing training emphasizes perfect form.

Years ago, during his "brute force" phase, Al usually did 50–60 full force throws in a practice session. Today, Al feels that his practice sessions are much more intelligently thought out. His maximum number of throws is 35 (he usually does less), with perhaps 70 percent at full force. However, because he is working on perfecting his technique, these sessions are much more productive than those earlier in his career.

Al feels that some aerobic training is important for cardio-vascular health and general conditioning, but he doesn't overdo aerobics. He does about three aerobic sessions per week of about 25–30 minutes on a cycle ergometer. This amount of work is about the right amount for fitness without cutting into strength and throwing ability, and he has found that indoor cycling is more convenient and interesting than jogging.

This overall schedule has worked terrifically well for Al. Except for an almost accidental injury, which unfortunately occurred right before the 1984 Olympics, Al has been virtually injury-free during this "second season" of his athletic career. In the 1968 games, Al threw the discus 212'6". In 1980, Al's best throw was 227'11". Prior to the 1984 Olympics, Al was up to the two-teens. For the next two years, Al focused on background and technique work and was throwing about 205'. Al planned 1987 to be a conservative year on the way to peaking in 1988 when he hopes to be in the 210' to 215' range, a distance that should put him in the Olympic Trials.

Some of the "secrets" of longevity common to other top masters athletes are found in Al's techniques and overall training approach. First and foremost, his training is interesting and enjoyable (more about this later). He takes long periods of time to round into top, peak shape; then backs off and builds up again (see Chapter 3). The volume, intensity, and duration of his training have evolved over the years to levels that are ideally suited to him. Each session and phase has a specific purpose. For example, rather than wearing himself down on hard throwing sessions which may be characterized as "heaving" sessions, Al's throwing sessions are shorter and more focused on technique. Injury is less likely to occur in such sessions and recovery is easier, yet these sessions provide a much better and more efficient training stimulus. In a word, Al's training and that of other top masters athletes is more "intelligent" than their youthful efforts.

Training Environment and Life-Style

Virtually all the masters athletes featured in this book have made training and competition a major priority in their lives. Often considerable effort and resources are put into developing an optimal training schedule and environment. Al tends to follow this general observation and guideline, but with some interesting exceptions.

First, it is important to note that Al is retired. In actuality, it is more accurate to say that he has a second, more casual career. He is in great demand doing motivational speeches for various businesses and organizations and does promotional work for two large firms (the Reebok Corporation and Eagle Fitness Equipment) involved in different aspects of sports and fitness. These activities do take some real time and effort, but do not detract from his training and life-style.

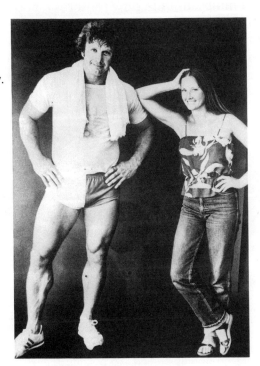

Al and Kathy.

Lest anyone believe that being able to reach such a position in life at a comparatively young age was easy, it must be noted that Al had a 25-year career with Grumman Data Systems. His primary work involved managing technical people (Al has a business administration degree from the University of Kansas), and to some extent he also was involved in the emerging computer technology during his tenure there (1959–1984).

In Al's earlier competition days, he kept at his work at Grumman and only took off vacation time before Olympic games. At that time, he had no elaborate sponsorship as some athletes enjoy today. Al is quick to point out, however, that he never sought time off and sponsorship. He reasoned that: "If I asked nothing of them, they could ask nothing of me." Then, and now, Al put a high value on his independence.

Al's training needs, both years ago and today, are very basic. Unlike some athletes, he does not have an entourage of trainers, coaches, doctors, and psychologists. As described above, his weight training schedule only requires a good, basic heavy gym—nothing fancy. He usually lifts alone with his wife, Cathy, as a spotter for heavy lifts. Rarely will Al work out with other power-lifters. For aerobics, he has his cycle ergometer. And his throwing usually only requires a high school field set up for track and field events.

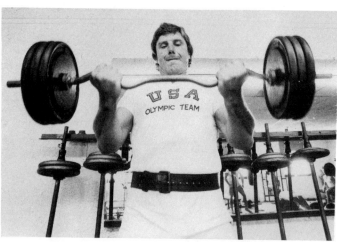

Al has no trouble curling 165 pounds in a workout.

Al spends six months of the year on Long Island and six months on the west coast of Florida. In both places, a gym and high school field are close to home. As one might also guess,

Al's life is not in the fast lane. When on Long Island, he takes advantage of the life-style afforded by the area—gardening, reading, using the beach, and visiting good seafood restaurants. He also is sure to spend as much time as possible with his grandson, a point we will return to shortly. In Florida, his life-style is similar, and he is able to spend time with his father.

This rather relaxed life-style is in contrast to his years at Grumman, particularly those when he was out of training. Al initially thought that would be his time to climb the corporate ladder. However, he found some of the pressure and politics involved in the climb not that suitable for him.

Perspective and Motivation

Many readers are doubtless wondering why Al stopped competing in 1968. Did he feel he had reached his physical limits? Was he burned out or injured? Actually, neither of these was true. At the time, Al was a single parent with two young daughters, and he felt that his best time and efforts should go into parenting. When his daughters became older, he started thinking about competing again. But he only did so when they gave their approval. Interestingly, Al said that it only took him a year to come back to good form and strength. This should be good news for readers who are either out of condition or simply have not trained hard for a while.

It can also be noted that on other matters, Al has always kept things in perspective. Over his long years of competition, he has learned that it's the process that counts. The outcomes— the awards and recognition—are great, but you really must enjoy the process. Or, as Al has commented, "It's always been the journey . . . It's being there" (quoted to George Vecsey, New York Times, 7/1/84). Thus, Al's disappointment in 1984 wasn't that he could not win another medal but that he could not enjoy the fun and challenges of the trials and games.

These perspectives on life and competition are important motivators for Al. He does enjoy the journey and makes it more interesting and enjoyable by setting a series of both short-term and long-term hard but reachable goals. Readers will recall that this is a prime motivational strategy discussed in Chapter 2. Al noted the great satisfaction that he takes in reaching goals. An example of Al's throwing goals is shown in Table 4.

TABLE 4

AL OERTER'S THROWING GOALS*

Year	Goal	Comments	Achievement
1977	170'	If achieved, it meant he had carved out of his schedule the daily time and was relatively injury-free.	175'
1978	190'	If achieved, it meant he had regained most of strength, technique, and competitive edge of 1968.	205'
1979	210'	If achieved, it meant that he was a serious Olympic challenger, especially if training improved and energy flow was easy.	219'
1980	220'	If achieved, he would possibly have an Olympic spot and again be a world class competitor, especially if he remained injury-free.	227'

*All goals to be achieved without drugs, coaches, or a need to recapture the past.

Several points about these goals are particularly important. First, they were set just prior to Al's return to training in 1976. Second, the goals represented a step-by-step progression to reach the top again. Third, they were what I have called "hard but reachable goals." And fourth, Al has successfully used a similar goal-setting process in his personal and professional life.

In recent years, Al has been frequently asked to describe his personal standards or what he is ultimately striving for. Al's response is very down-to-earth and consistent with his overall views. Al does not have a perception of himself as a great Olympic champion (which, of course, he is), nor is he somehow trying to recapture his youth or use his remarkable athletic career as a way to become rich. Rather, he simply sees himself as trying in the most thoughtful and purposeful way to get to the next Olympics, and in the process, to experience the fun, challenges, and "joy of extending himself." He also admits to a fascination in seeing what it is possible to do at his age. At this point, except for some longer time required to recover from injuries, Al reports no noticeable signs of aging. He has never had any serious doubts about his training regime or abilities now or in the past. He analyzes subpar training and performances and makes changes without the depression and psychic agony reported by many athletes. Most of all, his training remains very satisfying, and Al feels that with his physical self under control, everything else in life is much more manageable.

Clearly, Al could see a time when he would no longer be able to train and compete at a high level. But in a statement that echoes the sentiments of many dedicated masters athletes, Al said, "I will train to the day I die."

BILL PEARL

The Early Years

For anyone involved in weight training and bodybuilding in the 1950s and 1960s, there were a few top men whom everyone admired. John Grimek combined strength, muscularity, and grace to a degree that has hardly ever been equalled and certainly not surpassed. Steve Reeves was the epitome of balance and symmetry, qualities often lacking in contemporary bodybuilders. Stars in the 1960s and 1970s such as Arnold Schwarzenegger attempted to integrate the qualities of Grimek and Reeves. Although Arnold achieved lasting fame in bodybuilding as one of the all-time greats, he never quite put together the ultimate combination—muscular size, definition, balanced proportions, and athletic grace. And it can be safely said that even contemporary stars—for example, Mr. Olympia, Lee Haney—while more defined than men from the prior decades, are still searching for that ultimate elusive combination.

However, for those of us who have followed the "iron game" for many years, there is one man who did come as close

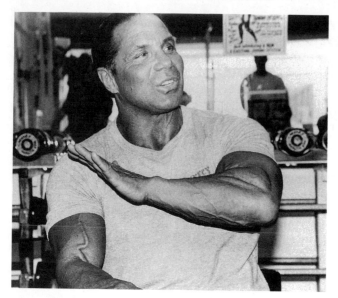

Bill looks
great just
sitting and
talking.

as humanly possible to perfection. His name is Bill Pearl. Today, in his late 50s, Bill is still in top condition and quite possibly is still the best.

William Arnold Pearl was born in Prineville, Oregon, in Oc-
tober 1930. Bill is a Nez Percé Indian and primarily grew up
around the Yakima, Washington, area. At the age of eight, Bill
saw an impressive strongman in a circus and decided that he
too wanted to be a bodybuilder and weightlifter. With determination, hard work, and goal directedness—characteristics
that have marked his entire life—Bill set out at the age of 11 to
become a strongman. Bill's father owned a restaurant, and Bill
trained by using gallon cans of vegetables as dumbbells and
gunnysacks of potatoes as a barbell. Training, even then,
wasn't haphazard. Bill kept records of his accomplishments
with the cans and sacks and systematically tried to surpass
them. After Bill's father sold the restaurant, the makeshift
weight equipment was left behind. It was replaced by hard
manual labor. Summer work in lumberyards and construction
sites became a way to earn some money and build muscle at
the same time.

Another major turning point occurred when Bill was 14. His

best friend, Al Simmons, had acquired a copy of the magazine *Strength and Health*, put out by the York Barbell Company. Together with another friend, the three boys scraped together about $40 and sent off for the basic York 110-pound set. However, because of the iron shortage in the war years, the boys had to wait for almost a year before the set arrived.

The boys set up a small gym in Bill's basement and agreed to train together every other day for an hour. Soon the other two boys lost interest in training, but Bill carried on alone, following the training courses that were included with the set. Bill added other plates, springs, grippers, and a crude bench to his home gym. He continued to religiously train during football, track, wrestling, and swimming seasons, at a time when weight training for sports was frowned upon. Thus, Bill was quite possibly the first weight-trained, all-around athlete.

Bill had numerous offers of athletic scholarships to colleges, but some critical events intervened. While traveling to visit his brother after high school graduation, Bill stopped off at the YMCA in Sacramento, California. The Y was then a hotbed of weightlifters and bodybuilders with one of the best training facilities in the country. Among the group of athletes was Tommy Kono, who went on to become a world record holder and Olympic weightlifting champion. In the workout that Bill observed, Kono was using weights that even by today's standards are incomparable (e.g., using two 110-pound dumbbells for standing military presses although he only weighed in the 140s). After the workout, Kono hit some incredible poses. Bill was overwhelmed and inspired, and as he said, "What I had seen had given me a vision of the future and the incentive to work even harder."

After this inspiring visit, Bill returned home with every intention of accepting one of his athletic scholarship offers. However, he ended up enlisting and serving in the Navy for four years. He first served on an island off the coast of Washington and then after two years was transferred to a station adjacent to San Diego. This transfer proved to be the single most pivotal event of Bill's adult life.

In San Diego, Bill met Leo Stern, a gym operator who had

trained some outstanding bodybuilders including Clancy Ross, the 1942 Mr. America. Leo quickly took Bill under his wing. He not only taught Bill how to train correctly and prepare for physique competition, but also how to set step-by-step goals in life (to be described later). And he showed Bill the ins and outs of successful gym ownership.

As they say, the rest is history. Bill won the series of titles listed below, became a legend in the sport, and owned a number of successful gyms in Sacramento and Los Angeles.

Bill in his late fifties looks terrific in one of his classic poses.

BILL PEARL'S PHYSIQUE TITLES

Year	Title
1953	Mr. Southern California
1953	Mr. California
1953	Mr. America
1953	Mr. Universe
1956	Mr. USA
1956	Mr. Universe (tall class)
1961	Mr. Universe
1967	Mr. Universe
1971	Mr. Universe

It is instructive to note that Bill won his last major title when he was over 40. However, the transitions in Bill's life during the last 10 to 15 years in many ways is more inspirational than his accomplishments in his younger years.

Life-Style Changes in Middle Age

After Bill's illustrious bodybuilding career, it would have been easy to slack off on his training and reap profits from his gyms, bodybuilding courses, consulting, and seminars. What is most intriguing and exciting about Bill is that he has never rested on his laurels—he has kept evolving and growing through his 40s and 50s. However, if truth be told, some of these changes were almost forced upon him.

In his book, *Getting Stronger*, (Shelter Publications, Inc., 1986) Bill recounted exactly where he was just prior to the "big 4-0":

> I was a three-time Mr. Universe winner lying on the couch in my living room, having a hard time clenching my fists and wondering what other medication I could take for the pain in my elbow and knee joints. I also had high blood pressure, high cholesterol and high uric acid.

Bill's deteriorating health was finally making it difficult to train at a level necessary for a world-class bodybuilder. It was also ironic that at this time Bill was a consultant training top executives and American astronauts. While he was rigorously training others and persuading them to adopt a healthier lifestyle, his own cholesterol count was 309! Visits with two doctors convinced him that he was a mortality statistic waiting to happen:

> It took this kind of scare to make me realize what I was doing. You generally think it will happen to the other guy and not yourself, but I realized I was just as vulnerable as anyone. Just because I was Mr. Universe and had a 19" arm didn't mean that I was healthy.

Bill's doctor had advised him to cut back on animal fats and sugar. Over time, Bill and his wife Judy did some serious study of nutrition and gradually made changes in their diet. They are now lacto-ovo-vegetarians, which means that they eat a vegetarian diet plus some dairy products and eggs. Bill feels that every year he has been following this sound nutritional approach, he has felt better both physically and psychologically. Interestingly, most modern bodybuilders have gotten away from the meat and protein onslaught of the 1950s and 1960s and have followed Bill's example in nutrition.

Another major change in life-style occurred somewhat later. Although Bill's businesses in Los Angeles were very successful, the long hours and pressure were starting to take their toll. During this time (mid-1970s), the fitness revolution was germinating, and Bill and Judy thought of an interesting and potentially profitable idea. Bill could not possibly train enough people personally to have an impact on the fitness boom. At the same time they noted that the training books that were appearing approached the subject piecemeal. Bill and Judy's original idea was to develop a comprehensive book on weight training and couple it with a personalized training program from Bill. Both the book and program would be sold through a mail-order business, perhaps helping to replace the hectic gym business.

Bill and Judy originally thought that the book project would take them about six months. However, they soon decided that instead of just showing and explaining a number of different exercises and variations, they would illustrate *every conceivable exercise on every piece of equipment*. The six months grew to four years plus the investment of over $200,000 of their own money.

The result of their efforts was a 638-page five-pound book, with over 3,000 illustrations, entitled *Keys to the Inner Universe: An Encyclopedia on Weight Training*. Bill and Judy took a chance and initially had 10,000 copies made. They sold the book through their mail-order business together with personalized training courses.

Eventually it became impossible to keep up with the number of requests for personalized training, and the large and expensive book was selling surprisingly well. Bill became convinced that the book could be sold wholesale through health and weight training stores. By this time the original book had sold 70,000 in softcover and 15,000 in hardback.

In the early 1980s, Bill realized that the interest in fitness and weight training was growing at a phenomenal rate and that he could play an important role in this development. The *Keys* book had only focused on bodybuilding, not the more general use of weight training for sports and general fitness and conditioning. Clearly, a book focusing on these more broad uses of weight training could have a substantial market. The result of this insight is Bill's book, done in collaboration with Gary Moran, entitled *Getting Stronger*. This is also a large, encyclopedic book that is written in a clear, concise, and interesting way. Despite being published by a small firm, the book is becoming one of the largest sellers in this field.

During the development of Bill's first book, he and Judy made another major life-style change. They moved from Los Angeles to a small town near Medford, Oregon. They bought a small ranch, and Bill converted an old barn into his personal gym. The area has proven to be a perfect place to have a relaxed life-style, yet at the same time has allowed Bill to actually expand many of his business interests. Today, besides his books, Bill is involved in marketing health foods and gym equipment, operating a health food store, and giving lectures and seminars around the country.

As we have seen in this book, the lives of many masters athletes have continued to evolve in interesting ways in their middle years. This is certainly the case with Bill, but with two exceptions: his training and goal-setting strategy have remained remarkably stable.

Training and Motivation

More than 30 years ago, Bill developed an approach to training that he found uniquely suited him. While Bill has been and is always willing to experiment with different methods and equipment, his basic approach has remained the same.

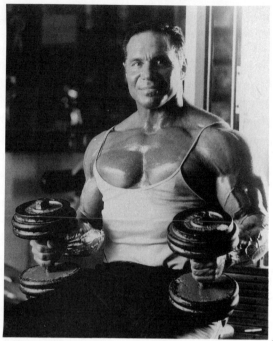

Bill looks unreal in this training shot.

Bill's training program is best described by such terms as very high volume and duration, moderate intensity, and considerable variability. In a typical routine, Bill will do several different exercises per body part for three to five sets each. This adds up to anywhere between 10–20 sets per body part. Bill most often uses a split routine, alternating training days for upper and lower body. Most of the weights he uses are about 85–90 percent of maximum (for the given repetitions and weight). Thus he rarely trains to failure and virtually never burns out.

Bill has always emphasized strict form and only short rest periods between sets. He reports that by following this training style, he can still use very respectable weights while managing to keep his heart rate at between 70–75 percent of maximum for extended periods. In a sense, his weight workouts are a form of interval training. Interestingly, circuit weight training, which tends to use lower weights, has been shown to have some (minimal) aerobic effects. It could be that Bill's approach is *more effective* for strength, bodybuilding, and aerobic benefits.

In more recent years Bill has added about 30 minutes of rowing and indoor cycling to his upper and lower body workouts respectively. Bill also changes his training routine every four to six weeks. Overall, his training occupies about two and a half to three hours per day.

Bill has noticed in recent years some possible effects of aging. His elbows and knees are sometimes stiff and a bit tender. When he gets up in the morning, his lower back is often stiff. Bill has learned to deal with these problems in two ways. First, he is no longer that concerned with pushing maximum weights in workouts. Second, he takes much more time to warm up. Besides his 30 minutes of aerobics, Bill does other exercises and abdominal work prior to his bodybuilding. Thus, his warm-up lasts about 45 minutes.

One major aspect of his training has not changed. Over the years, Bill has adapted to a schedule on which he goes to bed at 8:00 P.M. and is up by 3:00 A.M. After some herbal tea, fruit, and a bit of quiet time, Bill is ready to start his warm-up and aerobics at 3:45. At 4:30, he is frequently joined by his wife, Judy, a visitor or two, and one or more training partners. They all follow Bill's routine, and finish their workouts by about 7:00 A.M. After breakfast, Bill's eight- or nine-hour workday begins.

For some people, even the most dedicated of athletes, this schedule, which is followed six days per week, would become an ordeal. Bill, however, thrives on it and rarely misses any training days.

To keep himself motivated, Bill does many of the things that other athletes do. For example, he always keeps records of all his workouts and uses this as a comparison base for his present efforts. He sets both short- and long-term goals, a process we will examine in detail in a moment. He also has set up almost a perfect training environment for himself. This includes having a great gym at his disposal and being able to fine-tune his schedule for training. As we noted in Chapter 2, being able to set up an environment highly conducive to training is one of the keys to long-term motivation and success—a factor that is intuitively obvious but often overlooked in motivational theories that only focus on "person"-centered variables. Clearly, however, environmental factors interact with personal factors.

Not surprisingly, Bill is a keen observer of his progress. He formally and informally monitors his appearance, body weight, workouts, energy level, and recovery. He adjusts his training and life-style based on these continuous observations. But Bill's personal standards have not wavered over the years. His personal standard is still to be the best athlete and the best human being that he can be. He still sees himself as a model or example that others may be inspired to follow. The environment that Bill has established allows these standards and behaviors to come to fruition.

Goal-Setting

Goal-setting is a key motivational strategy (see Chapter 2), and one that Bill has elaborated upon:

> Regarding goals that I set for myself, here is an example. I will get a project like my new book, *Getting Stronger*, started. I know I am going to have to get in condition for photos in the book, so I will concentrate on this as if I was back in competition. I will also set up some personal appearances (such as posing exhibitions) so that I know I will have to be in condition for them. I will then do everything in my power to get in the best possible condition.

Essentially, Bill has been able to set long-term goals, and then backtrack and set up motivational steps along the way to his ultimate goal. He also is careful to avoid projects that he is not completely convinced will be beneficial. In the event that he is involved in a less-than-successful project, he will still put in great efforts to make sure the project bears at least some fruit. In addition, he has the satisfaction of having put forth maximum effort.

The Future

As Bill has gotten older, his example has become inspirational to more people. This is because he has reached a much wider audience through the sale of his books. He is now becoming an important role model for more senior citizens, middle-aged athletes, "youngsters" in their 20s and 30s, and even teenagers. Bill's present goal is to have an impact on our country's aging population. He hopes to do this possibly through another book project aimed at providing material on exercise, nutrition, and motivation to middle-aged and older Americans. This project may take him two to three years, and it will be interesting to observe the steps along the way to attaining his goal.

In the long run, Bill will use two other rich sources of motivation. First is the example and philosophy of his father, who is still going strong at 85. His father feels that every day should be used to produce or attain something of value. This can be as simple as mowing the lawn or as complex as starting an involved project.

Since Bill indicated that projecting an appropriate image and being an inspirational model are very important to him and help fuel his motivation and training, we will likely find Bill just as enthusiastic and training just as constantly and hard 20 years from now!

LYNNE PIRIE

At 38, Dr. Lynne Pirie is the youngest athlete featured in the portrait section of this book. Therefore, it is not surprising that she has been facing one of those challenging crossroads of her life, a point reached and traveled through by many of the athletes featured here.

In the late 1970s and early 1980s, Lynne was a role model for many women. Her astounding physique gave her such prestigious bodybuilding titles as "Miss USA 1982" and allowed her to compete at the highest professional level in 1985, the Ms. Olympia contest. During this period, Lynne was working on a

Ph.D. in Exercise Physiology and Growth and Development and completed the requirements for her D.O. degree in osteopathic medicine, with both sets of studies done at the highly selective Michigan State University.

During the last few years, Lynne has set up a busy practice as a physician and surgeon specializing in sports medicine and family practice. She has authored a highly successful training and fitness book, is a broadcaster for women's bodybuilding events, has her own weekly TV show, and does promotional work for commercial concerns. In addition, Lynne devotes some of her time to public service. She has been active in Muscular Dystrophy and Children's Hospital telethons.

Her schedule provides enough work and challenges for two people, but there has been a recent addition to her life. In March 1987, a daughter, Sarah Diana, was born to Lynne and her husband, John Schmelzer. And, thus, Lynne has reached the proverbial crossroads. Lynne is still young, is genetically gifted for her sport, and can generate incredible degrees of self-discipline—all qualities that could put her at the top again in bodybuilding. However, her family and work responsibilities preclude competition-level training at this point in her life. And, as Lynne explained to me, in bodybuilding and most other sports, once you have competed at the top, you cannot go back and compete at lower levels.

While it is not entirely clear how Lynne's life will evolve over the next several years, describing her past training and accomplishments and how she is meeting her new challenges should be instructive.

Background

Besides being an excellent student in high school and college, Lynne was also an outstanding athlete. Her first sports were basketball and track and field. In high school, Lynne was extremely versatile, running the 440, high jumping, and shot-putting. Later in college, and for a few years thereafter, Lynne specialized in the 800- and 1,500-meter runs. Her best times were 2:12 for 800 meters and 5:20 for the 1,500.

Lynne began bodybuilding in 1978 and at that point

Despite her family responsibilities and busy medical practice, Lynne looks terrific at thirty-eight.

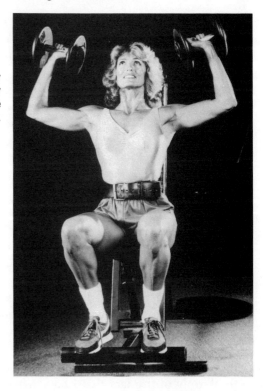

dropped competitive track. Lynne does continue to run for fitness and weight control, but at a reduced intensity from her competitive days.

Lynne did not have the most auspicious beginning to her competitive bodybuilding, but this tale says a lot about her:

> I loved to train with weights ever since my college basketball coach introduced them to me in 1969. That summer I joined "Jim's Gym" in my hometown and began to develop calves—that drew stares! I continued to do 20- to 30-minute workouts three times a week most of the time. Then when track stopped, I wanted to do something "intense" for my leg muscles—since I wouldn't be sprinting much—so I increased the weights. Soon there was a bodybuilding contest for women—"The Best in the World"—in a small town near Philadelphia. I was sure I could win, so I entered, didn't even finish in the top 12! But my

training partner, who I had *started* in bodybuilding, took First
Place! I was furious—happy for her, but *mad* for me—so I went
back and trained twice as hard—by *myself.*

After intensifying her training, Lynne started to see results and
realized that she had unusual potential for the sport. She soon
set as her goals achievements that ordinarily would take most
bodybuilders 10 to 15 years or more to fulfill: to win a national
title and compete professionally at the highest (Olympia)
level. Lynne achieved those goals in four and seven years,
respectively, while at the same time completing her rigorous
academic and medical education!

Lynne credits her disciplined upbringing with giving her the
skills to organize her life and achieve what others consider
impossible. Lynne described how she trained for contests:

> I would set a goal and then discipline myself through every
> detail, including diet, workout, tanning sessions, and time de-
> voted to developing my (posing) routine. I would schedule
> each of these events, and I would doggedly achieve each of
> them on schedule. I would let nothing get in the way. I would
> think only of the fact that I had to achieve what I had written
> down to achieve.

Of course, at the same time she was devoted to medicine and
her patients. Lynne explained that she would simply arrange
her schedule to meet all her training and medical responsibilities, including emergencies. Lynne is the first to admit that this
extraordinarily disciplined life had some costs. For example,
except for rare weekends, she had little or no social life.
Lynne's typical day's schedule shows what "discipline" meant
during her competitive days.

Competitive Philosophy and Motivation

Lynne did not emulate other female bodybuilders or athletes;
she did not have a particular female role model. Interestingly,
however, Lynne noted that Arnold Schwarzenegger influ-

TABLE 6

COMBINING COMPETITIVE BODYBUILDING WITH A MEDICAL CAREER

5:30 A.M.	Awaken; run or ride bike for 30 minutes; shower; breakfast
6:30 A.M.	Leave for hospital
7:00 A.M.	Rounds at hospital with most serious patients
7:30 A.M.	Surgery; see emergency room patients or read between cases (time out somewhere for lunch)
2:30 P.M.	Surgery and/or patient rounds
4:30 P.M.	Rounds with patients for next day's surgery
6:30 P.M.	Bodybuilding training for 2½ to 3 hours
9:30 P.M.	Eat, relax
10:00 P.M.	Read technical and other material
11:30 P.M.	Sleep

enced her most as a bodybuilder. She did not want to look like Arnold, but was (and still is) very inspired by his self-discipline and motivation, qualities in Arnold that Lynne feels are exemplary, matched by no one else, and certainly worth modeling. She also heartily agrees with Arnold's philosophy that he cultivated in the earlier part of his career: bodybuilding (or any other sport) should not be your entire life, only part of it. The sport should be blended into other parts of your life so as to enhance these different facets of life. However, Lynne is quick to point out that this perspective does *not* mean that you slight the sport because it is one of a number of things you do.

It is correct to say that during Lynne's competitive days, bodybuilding often was a major focus of her life. It is instructive to look at the major motivational strategies Lynne used then and later see how she uses these and similar strategies today.

We have already seen how Lynne would make an exact plan of her activities each day, structure a schedule, and doggedly stick to it. Lynne also had other techniques when she was competitive.

Personal Standards Lynne's personal standards for excellence were (and are) extremely high but realistic. These standards included being consistent, continually improving in training, never missing workouts, and being as physically and psychologically prepared for contests as is humanly possible.

Self Observation   Lynne found a very detailed training log, which provided a check-off list of all exercises completed, a record of her improvement, and tangible evidence of her consistency as the log became thicker over time. Lynne also regularly tracked her percentage of body fat and often compared her mirror image to pictures of herself at her best. The objectives here were to obtain a very low percent of body fat and surpass her previous best condition. Her coach, Jerry Doyle, also closely tracked her training and appearance.

Self-Evaluation   Lynne invested considerable thought and emotion in meeting and exceeding her goals and standards. Her exceptional performances led to feelings of elation and self-statements about personal worth and efficacy. Conversely, when she failed to meet or exceed standards or goals, she often felt depressed. Neither high nor low periods resulted in tangible instances of self-reward or punishment, although Lynne's behavior toward others varied from "gregariousness and extroversion" to being "humble and subdued." Most importantly, when faced with (perceived) failure, Lynne was able to have a "good introspective exam," figure out what went wrong, and develop the "quiet resolve" to come back stronger than ever.

Self-Efficacy and Outcome Expectancies   Except at the end of her competition days when her work responsibilities became extremely heavy, Lynne's belief in her abilities and her training program were always extremely high. Of course, these beliefs were fueled by her exceptional performances which, in turn, resulted in stronger beliefs and performances in the reciprocal influence process described in Chapter 2.

External Factors   Lynne has had a long relationship with a personal coach who always kept her on track and provided encouragement and feedback. Lynne described Jerry Doyle as "just like a father," someone she could absolutely trust. In his youth, Jerry, a competitive diver and acrobat, was one of the first athletes to use weights to enhance his performance. Jerry had unusual muscular potential, and if he were a young man today, Jerry would be a top bodybuilder. In his 60s, Jerry took Lynne under his wing. As Lynne explains:

> Jerry trained me for free! He took me to contests and paid for everything. He was the kindest, most generous, yet motivating individual I have ever met. I trained hard because this former great champion was training me—and I really didn't think I was worth it—so I'd better work hard to become worthy of this type of attention.

Lynne also created a very motivational climate for herself by often making public commitments about winning certain contests. She was regularly featured in the Weider publications and received considerable encouragement from the International Federation of Bodybuilders to compete. While competing itself was not particularly financially rewarding, her fame did contribute to the success of her book and personal appearances. It also attracted more patients to her practice. Finally, as noted, Lynne was able to create and stick to a work and training schedule that was highly conducive to optimal performance in each arena.

The Present and Future

While Lynne's life when she was competing and her life now have been presented as quite different from each other, in actuality, the changes have been more evolving than abrupt. Once Lynne's work and family responsibilities started to increase, it became apparent that her goal of winning professional contests had to be altered. Her first modification of her goal was to replace winning with the goal of continuing to be able to compete at a professional level. This new goal lasted for about a year and was never very satisfying. After some introspection, Lynne realized that:

> There are many avenues for victory or success. Why waste time and effort just to be less than I was . . . so I retired and redirected my energy to bodybuilding for health, fitness, and appearance, not competition. I even took up tennis and golf.

However, Lynne continues to take her training very seriously. She still regularly monitors her percent of body fat and her appearance and records all her training exercises, weights, and repetitions. Her schedule is just as ambitious as ever. She trains five days per week from 6:00 A.M. to 8:00 A.M. in the Sports Fitness Center, which is part of the North Phoenix Health Institute where she works. The gym has a wide assortment of equipment and is designed for rehabilitation purposes as well as high-level strength and fitness training. After training, some days she works for nine hours, while two other days a week her work continues round the clock at the Urgent Care Center.

Despite her hectic schedule, Lynne has not completely given up the idea of someday returning to competition. She regularly reads bodybuilding magazines to check the appearance of her former rivals and new entrants to the scene. She feels that she is physically at about 80 percent of what she was when training for competition. Just because "others are no longer watching you on a stage does not mean you have to stop caring for yourself and striving."

By not competing and by redirecting her energies, Lynne has found new areas of opportunity. From the mass media perspective, she is more appealing now than in her competitive days. This is because while bodybuilding has become quite popular, an all-around sportswoman is still a more acceptable and promotable image. Thus it appears possible that Lynne may have more impact in the media now that she is no longer competing. The popularity of her TV show, "Fitness First," attests to her impact.

Not surprisingly, Lynne's practice is thriving. At this point, Lynne is in constant demand both as an attending physician and as a lecturer. Her practice is now about 75 percent sports medicine and about 25 percent family medicine. Her TV work has expanded so that topics now include health, medicine, some news, and inserts for other programming, as well as fitness.

Lynne's first venture into book writing was also a success. *Getting Built!* (Warner, 1984), a complete bodybuilding and

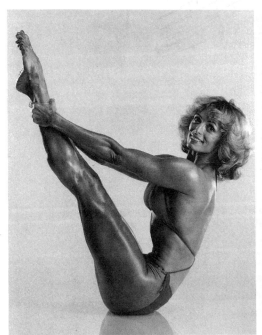 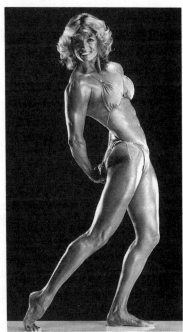

These pictures show why Lynne may successfully return to competition.

fitness guide for women from the novice to the competitive athlete, has sold over 80,000 copies. Her second book is called *Pregnancy and Sports Fitness* (Fisher Books, 1987). It comprehensively reviews what is known about pregnancy and exercise and provides advice on how to modify training over the course of pregnancy. There are also specific programs for dealing with foot and back pain, preparing muscles for an easier delivery, and a program to get back into shape after delivery. The book covers 30 sports.

Three more books are in the preparation phase. Lynne is particularly motivated to get back into terrific shape for the photo sessions that accompany the production of each book.

With all her professional activities, Lynne is still able to give quality time to her daughter and husband—time that realistically would be difficult to find if she were competing. Thus, although some things have been lost, much appears to be gained by the new directions in Lynne's life.

In the next several years, Lynne wants to specialize professionally in muscular rehabilitation, particularly of the lower back. Her program has significantly helped many back-pain sufferers, and her facility is set up to work with many patients.

Perhaps what is most intriguing is that Lynne's multidimensional life, with success in personal and professional realms, could become a model for women (and men) to emulate in the 1990s.

BOBBI ROTHMAN

For anyone who has been training for a long time, learning about Bobbi Rothman will lead to some very intriguing "What if . . . ?" thoughts. And for those readers in their 30s and 40s who are not serious athletes, another set of "What if . . . ?" thoughts should be aroused.

Bobbi was born in September 1945, in Pittsfield, Massachusetts. She had a nonathletic childhood and adolescence. Her major love was music, and in 1967 Bobbi received a bachelors degree in music education from the New England Conservatory of Music. In 1974, Bobbi was awarded a masters degree, also in music education, from New York University. Bobbi was a public school music teacher for 20 years. She has recently retired from that profession and is now devoting her full-time attention to her training and business interests. Bobbi is also in demand both as a private music teacher and personal fitness trainer.

Bobbi did not start exercising regularly until she met her husband Hal in the early 1970s, and she did not start to seriously train until she was in her mid-30s. As we will shortly see, Bobbi is now one of the top masters runners in the country.

For the long-term athlete, Bobbi, who keeps improving each year, presents a powerful psychological challenge. What if you had no records or other yardsticks of your performance in your 20s and early 30s and, further, did not expect to have decreasing performances in your 40s? Is it possible you would go far beyond what you now perceive to be your limits? For the nonathlete, and even for the person who is not even exercising, Bobbi's example raises the question, "What if you started?" Since you have never really tried, no one knows your true potential.

Records and Training

After only eight years of serious training, Bobbi has set a number of outstanding personal records and run some incredible races. Table 7 lists her current personal records.

TABLE 7

Distance	Time	Year
Mile	5:24	1986
5K	17:44	1985
8K	28:32	1986
5 mile	28:55	1984
10K	36:08	1986
12K	44:26	1987
15K	55:10	1986
Half Marathon	1:19:56	1985
Marathon	2:43:36	1986

Bobbi's most notable races were the 1985 New York Marathon, the 1986 Boston Marathon, and the 1987 Lilac-Bloomsday 12K. In all three of these prestigious races, Bobbi was the first American masters runner, and she set an American age group record in the 12K race. She was also the winner of the Orange Bowl 10K in 1986; and in 1987, Bobbi was the first or second place master in over a dozen prestige races (e.g., Falmouth). Of course, virtually all her PRs and best races were achieved *after* the ripe old age of 40.

For all her serious training in recent years, her coach has been her husband, Hal 41, who was an outstanding 100, 220, and quarter-miler in high school and college. He achieved a 47.6 quarter while running for Brockport University. He went on to receive a masters degree in physical education from Syracuse University and then taught in public schools for 18

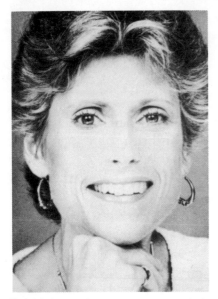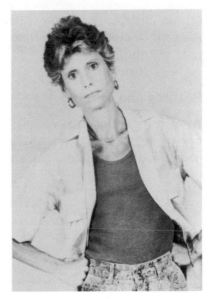

Bobbi shows that you can not only improve and run fast marathon times in your forties, but you can also look great.

years. While maintaining a very heavy and creative teaching load, he ran for the Long Island Athletic Club. He continued his prowess as a sprinter, doing a 9.6 for 100 yards and a 21.6 for the 220. These excellent times qualified him for the 1969 Maccabiah games.

Throughout the 1970s and early 1980s, Hal coached some outstanding teams and runners at the high school and college levels. Eventually, Hal turned his attention to longer distances and has a 32:05 10K and 2:43:00 marathon to his credit.

Currently, a good deal of Hal's energy is channelled into Bobbi's running career. He is her training partner and the architect of her overall program. Hal is also an account executive for Equity Planning, Barry Brown's agency.

Some key terms that can be used to describe Bobbi's training schedule are *instinctive* and *varied*. A lot of what she does is according to how her body feels on a given day. For example, if Bobbi feels tired, she does not feel guilty about taking an easy day. Conversely, if she's feeling particularly strong, she may take an especially hard workout. Her general goal is to get in three good-quality workouts per week, only one of which

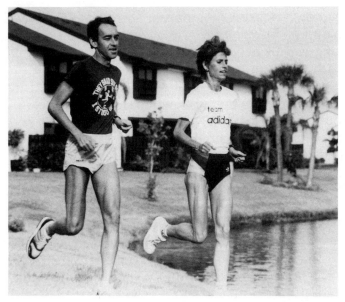

Bobbi with husband, coach, and training partner, Hal.

will be extremely hard. The hard workout is likely to be an interval workout or a race.

To help guide these decisions, Bobbi monitors her morning pulse, weight, and sleep. If her weight drops one or two pounds or her pulse is up more than four beats per minute, or her sleep was not restful, the training for that day may become a 30-minute jog or a day of complete rest. Thus, Bobbi closely monitors *recovery* (see Chapters 2 and 3).

The variety of Bobbi's training is best illustrated by looking in more depth at her training schedule. Twice per week, Bobbi does light upper body work, using a range of different movements and light dumbbells. Several times per week, she swims about a half mile, a practice that Bobbi has found adds to her overall conditioning and flexibility, with the bonus of being relaxing. Two to three times per week, she does drills (high knees, quick steps) using a water vest in the pool. On the days when Bobbi only runs once, it is likely that she will run in the pool as a second workout.

Generally, Bobbi averages about 75 miles per week with 90 as a maximum. Compared to many top runners, her approach is decidedly "relaxed." As noted, she spaces hard and easy days based on how she feels. In a week, Bobbi is likely to take one long run of between 90 and 120 minutes at a 7:00–7:20 pace, a fartlek run, an interval session focusing on short repeats at a fast pace, and several easier runs on grass. There also may be three days in the week when she does double running workouts, or two double workout days and a race.

Her fartlek runs are almost never the same. Sometimes, for example, these runs will be done on a golf course, running the fairway, then jogging to the next one. Her interval session can also be varied, and she usually does not run on a track, but in a park. A workout may be six three-minute runs with a two-minute interval jog, or 12 one-minute runs with a one-minute interval jog. Her easy runs, Bobbi noted, are very easy and relaxed, about 30–45 minutes at a "conversational" pace. Very often, she added, Hal and Bobbi will only run for time (minutes) rather than distance.

A sample training program for a week is shown in Table 8.

TABLE 8

SAMPLE WEEK FROM BOBBI ROTHMAN'S TRAINING LOG

Day	Time	Description	Distance
Monday pulse: 43 wt: 104 sleep: 7½	A.M.	40-min. easy run with Hal; on grass; at about 7:15 pace; 62°, nice and cool	about 5.5 miles
	P.M.	45-min. run with training group; started at 7:20 pace and ended at about 6:00 pace *Note:* wore Grete Waitz Adidas Shoes	about 7 miles
Tuesday pulse: 42 wt: 104.2 sleep: 8	A.M.	75 min. run with Hal in park; tired from P.M. run on Monday; very easy pace. *Note:* wore Questars.	about 9.5 to 10 miles
	P.M.	ran in pool for 20 min. and stretched	

Day	Time	Description	Distance
Wednesday pulse: 42 wt: 104 sleep: 8	A.M.	30 min. easy, then 3 × 7 min. pick-ups at 10K pace with Hal; 3-min. intervals; jogged for 15 min. and totalled about 75 min; *Note:* wore Fire IIs.	about 9 to 10 miles
	P.M.	½-mi. swim and 20 min. of light dumbbell work	
Thursday pulse: 42	A.M.	55-min. steady run with Hal in the park; 60°	about 7.5 miles
wt: 104.3 sleep 8½	P.M.	20 min. at a fairly good pace *Note:* wore Fire Ils.	about 2.5 to 3 miles
Friday pulse: 43 wt: 104.5 sleep: 8	A.M.	relaxed run with Hal on grass; started at 7:30 and then picked up to maximum speed *Note:* wore Questars.	about 9.5 miles
	P.M.	½-mi. swim and 20-min. pool run	
Saturday pulse: 44 wt: 104.5 sleep: 8	A.M.	30-min. easy run; 10 × 1-min. pickups with 1-min. interval; jog 5 min.; 2 × 3 min. with 2-min. intervals; jog 10 min. *Note:* wore Comps.	about 10 miles
	P.M.	20 min. light dumbbell work; then relaxed at the beach	
Sunday pulse: 44 wt: 104.6 Sleep: 7½	A.M.	95-min. run over grass with Hal at 7:15–7:25 pace; easy run, but 64° and humid *Note:* wore Questars.	about 13 miles
	P.M.	relaxed; dinner out	
		Total:	about 70 to 75 miles

Note: chances in schedule for a race on Saturday; Thursday run once and Friday run easy for 30–40 minutes.

Motivation

Bobbi has been highly motivated over the past five years by a series of hard but reachable goals. In the early 1980s, a major goal was to qualify for the Olympic Trials. Bobbi came quite close, but her 2:51:38 for the marathon at that point was not fast enough to qualify. From 1985 to 1986, her major goals were

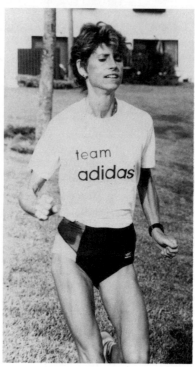

Bobbi warming up
for a relaxing run.

to break 37 minutes for the 10K and 29 minutes for five miles. She achieved both goals in 1986. For the last two years, her goals have centered on breaking 36 minutes for the 10K, qualifying for the Olympic Trial Marathon (which she accomplished with her 2:43:36 at Boston in 1986), and breaking the masters marathon record which is 2:39:11.

As discussed in Chapter 2, focusing on a series of hard, objectively defined, but reachable goals is a key motivational strategy. This approach is very different, and usually far more effective, than picking more nebulous goals such as "being a top masters runner." Of course, meeting specific goals provides the feedback and reinforcement necessary to sustain high-level efforts over long periods of time to meet another series of goals. Bobbi's success provides some nice documentation for the efficacy of goal-setting as a key motivational strategy.

However, while maintaining a focus on her goals, Bobbi still describes her overall perspective as "relaxed." She is not frantic about her training or future accomplishments. In fact, during training Bobbi visualizes herself running in a relaxed and relatively effortless way. Prior to competitions, she also visualizes herself running in a relaxed way over the course with her competitors.

Bobbi's strong relationship with Hal has played a critical part in sustaining her motivation. As we will shortly see, Bobbi has complete confidence in Hal's training programs. But moreover, Hal is her best friend, coach, and training partner—all these roles wrapped up in one person. Early on, Hal recognized Bobbi's potential and has been the guiding force in her success.

Bobbi is becoming sufficiently successful and recognized so that external reinforcement is becoming more prominent. She has been a member of Team Adidas, which means that she has received some equipment, along with a few trips to races each year. Although Bobbi cannot yet make an adequate income through racing, winning and prize money are nevertheless important reinforcers. Perhaps what is particularly important is the recognition she is receiving as a top runner. Bobbi has been featured on the cover of *The Runner*, and additional stories about her are regularly appearing in magazines and newspapers. She is becoming a role model for younger and older women by proving that a woman can be a top-flight athlete, yet maintain a loving relationship and be dynamic, articulate, and attractive. Of course, there is a real reciprocity involved in becoming a role model. The respect and adulation is wonderfully buoyant, but then there is the responsibility and hard work involved in living up to one's image.

Joan Benoit-Samuelson has been Bobbi's role model. Benoit-Samuelson has been at or near the top in American running for over a decade, and her triumph in the Olympic marathon was truly inspirational. But Bobbi notes that throughout all her success and recognition and even during noncompetitive times due to injury, Benoit-Samuelson has remained open and down-to-earth. These are qualities that Bobbi admires. Of course, at this point Bobbi is becoming a role model herself, particularly for younger women who admire her success and happy marriage. They are often surprised to hear Bobbi's age.

Another major factor contributing to Bobbi's motivation is the environment that she and Hal have created in Florida. At present, while Bobbi and Hal have an almost ideal training situation—and their daily schedule revolves around training—the environment has been created at some cost and risk. Some other masters athletes featured in this book have substantial income from other pursuits or receive financial rewards from their training, but that is not the case for Bobbi and Hal at this point. Thus, considerable commitment and risk have been involved in fostering an environment that will allow Bobbi to reach her ultimate potential as a masters runner.

Personal Processes

Since Bobbi directs a lot of her training and racing to meeting specific goals, it is not surprising that she keeps a very detailed training diary, as the table above shows. Bobbi not only records the time and approximate miles she runs in her workouts, but also how she felt in the session, the weather, the shoes she was wearing, and any other significant data. In addition, she also keeps track of all her nonrunning exercise and training sessions. Other data that she monitors on a daily basis are awakening pulse, hours of sleep, and her weight. Bobbi is not recording compulsively; she is gathering important data to fine-tune her workouts and to become part of her data base so that she can better understand variables associated with optimal training and peak performance.

Such intimate self-observations are also part of almost every workout. Bobbi can adjust workouts in progress or subsequent workouts based on her perception of her effort, her speed and endurance, and perhaps most important, her immediate and longer term recovery from particular workouts or a series of workouts. Bobbi is, therefore, one of the few athletes who has a systematic plan to monitor stress and recovery and *make changes in training and rest accordingly* (see Chapters 2 and 3).

If there is one word to describe Bobbi's overall approach,

the word is *disciplined*. Bobbi points out that parts of her disciplined (but, importantly, relaxed and not obsessive) approach are a carryover from the rigors of her music training. Fortunately, Bobbi's prior training and approach are excellent matches for Hal's training philosophy and strategies.

While there is nothing unusual about Bobbi's personal athletic standards ("To always do the best that I can"; "To try to get something out of every workout"), one point she made stands out as instructive to all athletes. It is important for Bobbi that she *enjoys* herself while training and competing. While she is very competitive and likes to win, personal relationships are really what are most important to her.

"Keeping things in perspective" is also part of Bobbi's self-evaluation of her training and racing. While she feels elated with good performances, she does not fall into the depths of depression following subpar performances. Instead, she reviews her performance, searches for the positive parts, and uses that information for planning future efforts.

Since Bobbi's training programs are so varied, fine-tuned, and specifically designed for her by Hal, she is very confident that the program she is following is the best possible one. Consequently, she rarely has been beset by doubts about the efficacy of her programs. Bobbi also acknowledges some natural ability as a runner and a high degree of confidence in her abilities. By far, though, she feels that her biggest assets are her discipline and tenacity. In fact, Bobbi commented: "I'm convinced that you do not need a lot of talent to be a competent and even outstanding runner."

Bobbi's example is inspirational to all middle-aged athletes (and would-be athletes). Not only can top performances be attained in the middle years, but improvement is also quite possible. A certain degree of natural ability is necessary to succeed at any athletic endeavor, but in the end, consistency and perseverance may be more important than "potential." Even so, success in athletics, even at the highest level, need not be equated with being obsessively driven or one-dimensional. Success as a person can come first and can complement success in athletics.

TODD SCULLY

Whenever I am out walking or riding around the Virginia Tech campus, morning, noon, or evening, I am almost always certain to see Todd Scully running, jogging, or walking. This man appears to be in perpetual motion—and, indeed, he almost is.

Clark Todd Scully, Jr. was born in Princeton, New Jersey, in September 1948, so he is one of our younger ageless athletes. Todd received his B.S. degree in chemistry from Lynchburg College in 1970, was in the Army from 1970 to 1972, and returned to Lynchburg College to receive a masters in education in 1974. From 1974 to 1976, Todd taught chemistry, earth science, and general math at Liberty High School in Bedford, Virginia.

Since 1976, Todd has been the distance running coach at Virginia Tech and the owner of two stores (the "Jock Shop") that primarily cater to runners. Todd is single, and most of his life revolves around coaching and his business.

Todd has had a distinguished career in track and field. However, as is the case with a number of other athletes featured in this book, many people in the community he resides in do not know or appreciate the level of performance Todd has achieved.

Records

Todd started seriously training when he was 16. For the next six years, he largely focused on running the half-mile and mile. Todd really hit his stride when he started race walking. His specialty has been the 20K and 50K distances. Todd made the U.S. Olympic team as a 20K race walker in both 1976 and 1980. He was on the 1975 and 1979 Pan Am teams, and on the World Championship team in 1973, 1979, 1981, 1983, and 1985. In 1979, Todd finished third in the 20K in the Pan Am games.

Between 1976 and 1980, Todd held the string of American and World records shown in Table 9. Recently, as a coach, Todd was named the Metro Conference Cross-Country Coach of the Year.

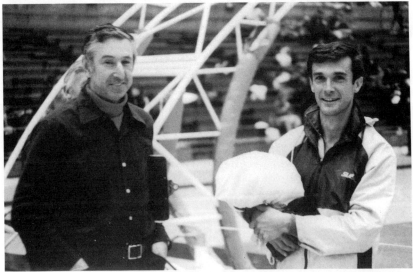

Todd with Elliot Deman, who helped him get started in race walking.

TABLE 9

TODD SCULLY'S RACE WALKING RECORDS

Year	American Distance	Time	Year	World Distance	Time
1978	1,500m	5:35.0	1978	1,500m	5:35.0
1978	1 mile	5:55.5	1978	1 mile	5:55.5
1978	3,000m	11:40.2			
1978	2 mile	12:35.0	1978	2 mile	12:35.0
1978	10K	42:29			
1979	20K	1:28.20			
1974	5,000m	21:04.3			
1977	3 mile	19:46.0			

Training

Like most of the other athletes featured in this book, Todd feels that he is still improving. He noted that he is stronger and faster now than ever before and capable of meeting or exceeding records he set a decade ago. Todd basically trains exactly as he always has over the last 20 years. He describes his approach as simply going as long and hard as possible. In practice, this means that three or four days per week he will do "relaxed distance" of about 15 miles. Two days are set aside for interval training, covering five to seven miles with repetitions faster than race pace. One day is used for overdistance training, with a session lasting between two and four hours. Thus, in Todd's schedule, there are two to three hard workouts per week, and he covers somewhat more than 100 miles each week.

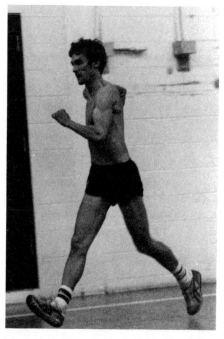

Todd works on his leg speed on the indoor track at Virginia Tech.

Since Todd has been training for so many years, he has a very long baseline to assess his current efforts. This means that for any specific workout, he can try to meet or exceed times he made years ago.

However, unlike when he was younger, Todd now only races infrequently. He has not been enticed by the many potential races; he prefers to do background workouts and then sharpen, peak, and taper for big races. This approach is much more the style of European athletes than Americans. Todd feels that American athletes often race too much and do not reach optimal performances. Todd will only maximally peak for the 1988 Olympic Trials and, at the same time, for a shot at many of the masters race walking records.

Todd's diet is similar to that of other endurance athletes—high complex carbohydrates—and he uses vitamin and mineral supplements. As for recovery ability, Todd feels that he recovers as well as he ever has from his high-intensity, high-volume training load. He has the usual assortment of aches, pains, and inflammations, but nothing that has interrupted his training. Indeed, he has not missed a workout in over 15 years!

Motivation

Todd feels that his motivation for training is much higher than ever before. He does not need to get up for a hard workout in any particular way. As a number of other athletes in this book have commented, simply planning and starting a hard workout is all the motivation Todd needs.

Todd seems purely motivated by the activity itself. He does not have training partners or coaches or belong to an athletic organization, and he does not feel that friends or peers play a role in keeping him motivated. While Todd's stores provide part of his income, few people seem to shop in them just because of his reputation. In fact, as noted before, few people know about his athletic achievements. Ironically, while he advocates using training logs as a coach, Todd does not keep detailed training records (only time for specific workouts), and he does not sell training diaries in his stores.

Similarly, Todd does not seek out feedback and reinforcement from other people. The only systematic feedback from others comes after high-level competition, when the judges and national coaches talk with Todd about his form. Nor does he seek any local or national media attention.

When Todd first started to seriously train for race walking, however, he did have a role model: he emulated the top person in the sport, who at the time was Ron Laird. Now, however, Todd is considered one of the top distance race walkers in the country, and essentially, he is his own role model. Todd is also now a role model for the athletes he coaches. I conjecture that "keeping up with the kids" and showing them he can still do it must be quite motivational.

Summarizing how he feels about his own motivation, Todd notes: "I am the sole mover in my motivation and I must do it from within, or I really don't want to do it." However, Todd admits that occasionally even his motivation has waxed and waned. His motivation has suffered when his work and coaching commitments became overextended. Todd also admits that once in a while he becomes bored with training and gets soft and lazy. Even during these down times, Todd never misses a training session. He just cuts back on his training intensity for a while. A new training goal or pointing toward a competition gets Todd started again in high gear.

Since Todd attributes most of his motivation to personal, internal processes, it is instructive to look at some details here about them. First, as has been noted, despite not using a detailed training log, Todd is a keen observer of his day-to-day performance. The key dimension for him is the time of specific workouts over certain courses. Pressing to meet or exceed previous times is particularly important as competitions become close at hand.

In competition, Todd has two "simple" self-standards: to win and do the best that he can. Since even Todd cannot always win, in reality the one major self-standard is to do the best that he possibly can on race day.

As with many masters athletes, regardless of competition level, subjective and objective performance appraisals can be emotional for Todd. When he meets or exceeds his goals, it leads to feelings of elation and (private) positive self-statements. When he fails to meet his goals, it often leads to more negative affect and even depression, particularly if he has prepared well for a workout or race. Thus, it is fairly easy to see how different feelings and self-statements can be very motivating.

Because of Todd's longevity, his approach has stood the test of time. He is "extremely confident" in his program and abili-

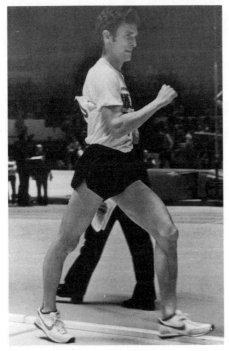

Todd on a record-setting pace
at Madison Square Garden.

ties. Only once did Todd doubt his approach, and that was when it was modified by coaches at the 1976 Olympic Trials. Todd feels his subpar performance was actually due to following the coaches' advice and *over-resting*. He actually had *too much energy* and could not properly pace himself!

Once in a while now, Todd has had some doubts about his abilities. A number of people have told him that he is getting too old for world-class performances. However, Todd has his current workouts to compare to his past efforts, which reaffirm his present abilities and race performance potential. In addition, Todd feels that the source of his performances and achievements has always been his terrific perseverance and determination, not great innate ability. If necessary, he is always willing to go harder and longer in his workouts—whatever it takes.

Environment

Todd's work schedule is reasonably flexible and the climate

and terrain around Virginia Tech and Blacksburg are quite suitable for training. However, for a person at Todd's level, conditions are not ideal. In other sports, including road running,
someone at the world or national level could earn a good
living just racing, or at most, working part-time. Todd essentially has three jobs: coaching, business, and training. Ideally,
Todd would like to work only part-time when he is training
very hard. In order to accommodate his work commitments, it
is not unusual for Todd to start a morning training session at
4:30 A.M. When training for a competition, things really become difficult. In order to accomplish all his training, Todd
cuts back a bit on sleep. The week before competition, all
other activities except training and sleeping become secondary. Another disadvantage is that Todd does not have ready
access to chiropractic and massage facilities, as do most other
world-class athletes.

Concluding Observations

In many ways, it is a bit sad and ironical to compare Todd's
status on campus to the lot of athletes in revenue-producing
sports. Many of these athletes are pampered and have some of
the best coaches and training facilities in the country at their
disposal. And, many of the athletes will stop being athletes as
soon as they leave the campus when their eligibility is completed. Todd, on the other hand, has been going it alone, at a
world-class level, but under much less than ideal circumstances, for almost a quarter of a century!

In briefly talking with Todd one day, I may have found one
critical ingredient to his longevity and steady improvement
into middle age. Todd said he always felt that aging was really
sociological and not physiological. He does not *expect* to
show inevitable decline. His training schedule reflects this belief, and if the recent past predicts the future, Todd will remain
a world-class athlete for many years to come, both in masters
and open competition.

TRACY SMITH

Many readers are probably familiar with Tracy Smith's return to world-class performances on the road and track. His background, training methods, motivators, and goals will be detailed shortly. However, one quote from Tracy summarizes the feelings and thoughts of many masters athletes who have returned to hard training or who never stopped training and competing and are always looking for new horizons:

> Most of the time I feel like a pioneer in breaking into new vistas of physical ability as an older athlete. That is a real motivator. To see just how close I can get to my world-class times of 15 to 20 years ago. Carlos Lopez, Antonio Villanueva, and Jack Foster have inspired me not to give up on trying to make new breakthroughs in distance running as a master runner!

Tracy was born in March 1945, in Pasadena, California. After high school, Tracy attended Oregon State from 1965 to 1966 and then California State University at Long Beach, where he received his B.S. degree in physical education in 1973. Tracy's most prominent positions after college were teaching in a continuation high school for six years and serving as a youth director for a Presbyterian church in Bishop, California, where Tracy continues to live. He was also a policeman for two years.

Tracy and Carolyn were married in 1974 and have three children: Ryan, who is 10; Jennifer, 7; and Erin, 5. Presently, Carolyn has a full-time job as a teacher, and Tracy is a full-time runner. His job now is to be the best masters distance runner in the world, and he helps support his family with money he earns racing and doing speaking engagements. Tracy is also sponsored by Reebok. They provide his shoes and running apparel and they pay his expenses to races.

Tracy is quick to point out that he takes his role as househusband very seriously. He considers that his full-time job. Many years ago, he and Carolyn decided that while their children were growing up, both of them would not work full-time outside their home. The Smiths want to devote as much time as possible to their children.

Except for three years when Tracy was in his early 30s, he has been a competitive runner since he started high school. He was fortunate, as we will see, to have good coaching at the

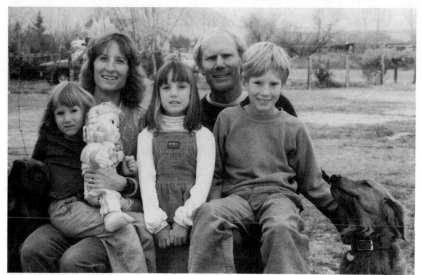

The Smith family: (front) Erin, Jennifer, Ryan; (rear) Carolyn, Tracy

outset. Indeed, Tracy's training today is an updated version of the methods he was taught and used 25 years ago.

When he started, Tracy first focused on cross-country (two miles) and the mile during track season. From 1964 to 1976, he primarily ran two- and three-milers and 10Ks, and from 1977 to 1985 he mostly ran 10K road races. Most recently, he has returned to his first love and best distance, the mile. And Tracy's success has been inspiring. As of this writing, he holds the world record for the masters mile and the American 10K masters road record. In Table 10, it can be seen that Tracy's records and accomplishments cover a remarkable 25 years.

Not surprisingly, Tracy's goals throughout his long career have paralleled his successes. First, his goals were to become the California state mile champion, aim for the 1968 Mexico Olympics, and break the American masters 10K record. Tracy's next goals are to break 4:10 for the mile or 3:52 for the 1,500 meters. Anyone who can consistently meet lofty goals has a good sense of their own talents and how to channel those talents and, in particular, in Tracy's case, an excellent training program and methods that over the years have been uniquely tailored to him.

TABLE 10

Year	Record/Accomplishment
1963	California State Mile Champion, 4:12.6
1966	3rd in the International Cross Country Race
1967	World Record Indoor 3 mile, 13:16.2
1968	World Record Indoor 3 mile, 13:15
1968	Olympic Trial Winner, 10K
1973	World Record Indoor 3 mile, 13:07.2
1987	World Record Masters Mile Indoors, 4:20
1987	National Masters Indoor Champion, 4:18.6
1987	American Record Masters 10K, 29:50

Training and Effects of Aging

Although Tracy may meet and even surpass some of his best race times of his 20s and 30s, he readily admits that his body does show some effects of aging. He has had some problems over the years with plantar fasciitis and now wears orthotics. A sciatic nerve condition comes and goes so Tracy does a good deal of stretching and is careful to have a proper build-up in his training and a warm-up in his workout before tackling speed work. He feels that his recovery between hard workouts is not quite as good as it was 10 to 15 years ago. Therefore, Tracy runs 50–60 miles per week these days compared to 80–100 miles per week years ago, runs only once per day, and sometimes takes two easy days between hard workouts. The repetitions in his interval training are also a little slower than in the past.

However, rather than seeing Tracy's current training as on the decline, if anything, his schedule appears better planned than his youthful approach and more in line with most of the basic points discussed in Chapter 3. Throughout his career, Tracy has relied a great deal on interval training, initially following the programs of Mihaly Igloi. What Tracy did in his youth would now be considered an example of overtraining. Tracy agrees that he probably overtrained when he was younger. But he feels that this was a very important part of his career, an absolutely necessary apprenticeship period. He also pointed out that the interval sessions were usually *not* timed, he was never injured, and these few hard years gave him a "mental toughness" that has been invaluable for high-level training and competition.

By his late 20s and early 30s, Tracy not only kept up some of his interval training, but also included road running and hill training at altitude. In his middle 30s, Tracy's running was mostly recreational and fitness-oriented and only included slow, steady runs of three to five miles four days a week. For his comeback, starting in 1981, Tracy went back to his interval training four days per week. He did not include any longer runs in his training, which Tracy now feels was a mistake.

Tracy's current schedule seems to be ideal for him, and probably would be for many other runners. He devotes three days per week to interval training, takes one long run that includes hills, and has two easy days. One day, usually Sunday, is completely a rest day.

Tracy has learned over the years to keep his training challenging and enjoyable; workouts are not to be dreaded (see Chapter 3), and he generally trains at a comfortable pace. However, these are by no means easy workouts. A week's worth of interval sessions is shown in Table 11.

TABLE 11

Day	Workout
1	8-mile run then 8 × 330 on grass and 1 × 1,320 on grass, all with a 110 jog in between and a 1-mile jog cooldown
3	12–16 × 440 at 68–70 seconds with 110 jog in between
6	Race simulation, 6 × 440 at 62 seconds with 110 jog in between

Motivation

Tracy provided an unusual amount of detail on sections of the questionnaire pertaining to motivation. Therefore, it is possible to obtain a rare glimpse of the many internal and external factors that come together in the making of a champion.

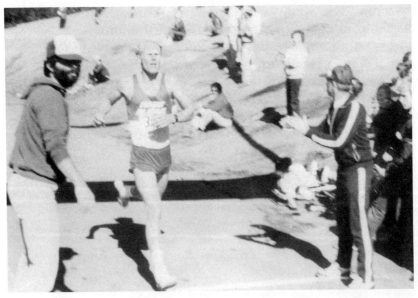

Tracy finishing strongly in a recent race.

Tracy's motivation for training and competition is just as high as it was 15 to 20 years ago, and certainly much higher than 5 to 10 years ago. A lot of his training, as we saw, is still directed to big interval sessions, and these successful sessions are the result of considerable planning and concentration. Almost all of Tracy's training is done very early in the morning so that there is maximum time and few, if any, distractions. He can give a big session days of prior thought and usually precedes it by two easy training days. Tracy also allows a good deal of time for the workout so that he does not feel stressed from time pressure. Yes, Tracy is a full-time runner, but because he takes his family, religious, and community responsibilities very seriously, training sessions, even super-hard ones, begin at 5:30 A.M.

If Tracy notices his desire for hard training waning, he varies his program. He will take advantage of the beautiful surroundings near Bishop and run on adventure trails for a few workouts. Tracy also limits his competitions to about one per month and has about a three-month period each year where his training is much more low-key. Thus, variety in his training, pointing to only a few key races, and having some down time each year help to keep Tracy motivated over the long haul.

Tracy's training includes a considerable amount of fast running and race simulations (see above table). These workouts prepare him well for competitions. Tracy feels that if he can do four excellent interval sessions in a month, he is ready for competition. His training and competition, as we will see, are also greatly aided by Tracy's strong religious beliefs.

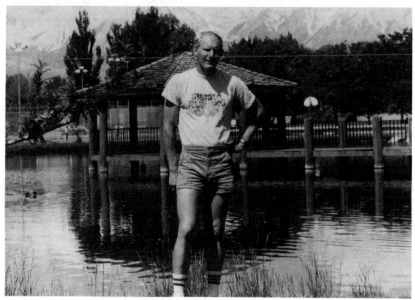

Just a look at this setting shows you why Tracy has settled in Bishop.

Other external factors play a strong role in Tracy's motivation for training and competing. Tracy does some of his training with his wife. Carolyn "pushes me out the door to train," and her pleasure in seeing Tracy excel is something Tracy also finds important. For many years, Tracy trained alone, but he now finds that having training partners for long runs is very valuable. Tracy can be described as "self-coached," but still corresponds with his high school coach, Bill Peck, for advice. The people of Bishop are extremely proud of Tracy's accomplishments, and Tracy feels very motivated by their interest and encouragement.

Tracy acknowledges that other external factors are equally

important. Although he loves competition and meeting new people and seeing new places, he realistically notes that he could not compete outside of Bishop without the financial returns of racing and the support of the Reebok Racing Team. He has enjoyed seeing himself featured in various running magazines. And, most certainly, the model of the "older" runner exemplified by Antonio Villanueva has provided Tracy with "the expanded vision that even at 46 and 47 a person can be competitive with the 40-year-olds."

Tracy, as we'll see shortly, also has a tremendous amount of confidence in his abilities. It is this confidence that has allowed him to make public statements and commitments about performances in races. For example, a week prior to the Crescent City Classic in New Orleans, he publicly said at the National Masters Indoor Championships that he would attempt to break Barry Brown's masters 10K mark. Tracy was able to fulfill this commitment; he bettered Brown's mark by seven seconds. Tracy finds that making such realistic commitments is also very motivating.

Tracy readily admits that he enjoys the attention he has been given by the local and national press, the positive publicity given to Bishop, California, and the surrounding areas, and the respect that he feels from peers as well as younger people. Even more important to him has been the opportunity to share his success with his wife and father and to use his new stature as a way to convey his religious faith to others. As Tracy notes:

> I want to be an influence in people's physical as well as spiritual life. They respect my physical ability and therefore respect my faith.

Tracy's extraordinary belief in his own abilities is matched by his deeply held religious beliefs. Tracy feels that his running ability is "the gift Jesus Christ has given me. He wants me to use it for His glory." Further, when Tracy does exceptionally well, he feels a special sense that "this is what God wants me to be doing because I can feel His pleasure at what I am doing." It is difficult to imagine being able to compete against someone with such a strong set of beliefs!

In addition to his religious beliefs, Tracy holds very lofty standards for himself and is an acute observer of his own behavior. Tracy does not just want to establish masters records *but also come as close as possible to the standards he set 15 to 20 years ago.* These standards include a 4:02 mile at 23, a 28:47 10K also when 23, and a 13:07 three-mile at 28. In his training, Tracy closely monitors (although without using a formal diary) all his workouts for time and intensity, his daily weight, and his ability to recover from hard workouts. He also tracks his time for intervals, endurance on long runs, running form, flexibility, and desire to run.

Each of these dimensions has specific markers. For speed, it is the ability to do many repetition 440s at 68 seconds or better. For endurance, it is the ability to feel good all day after running 15 or more miles in the morning. Form means feeling rhythmic and smooth when running. Flexibility is the ability to stretch as well as he did 15 to 20 years ago. Desire means looking forward to workouts and races and enjoying the entire process.

Tracy's personal standards for training involve being able to train hard nine months per year with three of those months centering on top performances. His goal is to compete well but, as noted before, only once per month. Each week in training, his basic goal is to run 50 to 60 miles with at least two good interval sessions and one long run.

For Tracy, good running performances are an affirmation of his faith. However, he does not become overly discouraged by poorer performances. He is most likely then to back off, take the pressure off himself, and just run for the joy of running.

As noted in the training section of this portrait, Tracy's program has evolved over the years into one that appears ideal for him. He is extremely confident in his program because time and time again it has provided the foundation for his great performances. He is also extremely confident in his abilities and knows that his competitive desire can usually take him further and quicker than even his best workouts would indicate. Indeed, since being able to train and compete full-time without being pressured by stress from his job or guilt from neglecting his family, Tracy feels "a new confidence and physical vigor."

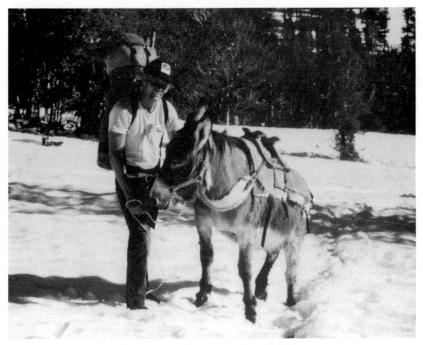

Enjoying some recreational hiking.

Tracy feels that his goals of closely matching the performances of his youth are within his reach. Yet he is realistic. He knows that without support he will not be able to train as well and certainly will not be able to compete everywhere. Tracy also knows that as the years go by, there may be some physical limitations that will make him no longer competitive with 40-year-olds. He feels that it would not be fair to his family then to continue to train and compete at such a high level.

When Tracy decides that his competitive days are over, he and Carolyn will probably become part of the Christian Mission Field. They both feel very strongly that their children should know firsthand about life in other countries that are not as affluent as the United States. Tracy also believes that his competitive drive will be channelled into "some other challenge in life to fulfill this desire to excel and serve God." Tracy and Carolyn want to do something that "we feel has eternal value in leading people to the Lord. I don't think there is any greater feeling of joy than that of being a servant of your fellow man."

HAROLENE WALTERS

For a variety of reasons, Harolene Walters was a late entry into the portrait section of this book. However, Harolene's inclusion is important. Her portrait nicely illustrates a number of the psychological and physical training principles at work in concert with each other. Harolene's approach and perspective on goal setting is illuminating:

> This year when I'm 45, I want to set some American age records and improve my 5K, 10K, and marathon times. And my big goal? I plan on running until I'm 100 years old!

Lest readers believe that such goal-setting is actually idle boasting, Harolene later noted that "I always set goals to achieve for myself. I generally never give up until I've achieved what I want to achieve."

More specifically, Harolene sees herself continuing to set American records in "older divisions." Her own assessment, which is certainly right, is that "there's no one my age at the present that I know of who can beat me." Harolene is aiming for setting a PR in the Olympic Marathon Trials, which she believes will also be an American age division (45–49) record. Harolene, however, is not just trying to "maintain" so that eventually records will come her way. She wants to improve her marathon time from 2:47:00 to 2:38:00, her 10K time from 36:18 to 36:00, and her 5K time from 17:30 to 17:15.

In reaching these times, Harolene will also be able to achieve another set of goals. She wants to become a "global runner," racing, for example, in London, Bermuda, and China. Harolene also noted that:

> These goals are picked because I feel that they are attainable. I channel my energy to meet these goals by being and feeling positive and training hard every day. And I love to win!

Background

Harolene cannot be considered a nonathlete who suddenly put on a pair of running shoes and within weeks discovered great latent aerobic power. Harolene does have an athletic background. In her early 20s, Harolene was a professional water skier in various water shows in different parts of the country. She also snow skied regularly and raced in downhill events. She kept up her water and snow skiing on a recreational basis into her early 30s. By her late 30s, Harolene was weight training for 45 minutes at a Nautilus gym three days per week and running five or six days a week. She also enjoyed biking and roller skating.

Harolene's favorite activity is travelling every summer; she has been to Asia, Africa, Europe, and South America. She collects antiques from all parts of the United States and has accumulated enough to open up an antique store. She loves to read when she has the time, but it's hard to find enough spare time in the day.

By the time Harolene was 40 she was racing occasionally, but her 10K time closely matched her age. Harolene was not yet training as a serious runner and did not pay much attention to nutrition. She was slightly heavy and not very muscular. As a result, her performances were not very notable. However, after she became more serious about her Nautilus workouts, she could see a big difference in how she felt physically as well as mentally. She felt better about her appearance and didn't have so much nervous energy. It's hardly surprising that Harolene decided to intensify her training.

Harolene is proof of the adage that, indeed, "life begins at 40." In a few short years, through a very tough training regime; good nutrition; and the advice, support, and coaching of her husband, Ron, Harolene has emerged as one of the top masters runners in the country. And she has reached the top in running while maintaining her full-time job as a special education teacher in the Los Angeles City School District, a position she has held for 15 years.

Training

Harolene's training is varied and well organized, as shown in Table 12 (p. 228). In examining her regime, one thought immediately came to mind. A few short years ago, very few people thought that anyone over 40 (much less a woman!) could train that hard.

TABLE 12

A TYPICAL TRAINING WEEK FOR HAROLENE WALTERS

Monday	10 miles at 7:45 pace
Tuesday	6 miles speed work and 3 × 1,000 meters
Wednesday	10 miles at 8:00 pace
Thursday	6 miles and a 3K time trial
Friday	8 miles easy and 6 × 200 meter relaxed strides
Saturday	6 miles easy
Sunday	20-mile long run

Harolene runs every day, from 50 to 80 miles a week depending on the event she will race. Her easier and moderate runs are done on bike paths near her home. Once or twice a week Harolene has a track workout. After a two-mile warm-up, she may do five-mile repeats, 1,320 six times or 800 eight times, or 400 twelve times, again depending on the event she is aiming for in the near future. All Harolene's repeats are run at race pace or better. The interval workout is followed by a one- or two-mile warm-down.

Once a week Harolene also will do a fartlek run on the roads with repeats and slower running times of from one to four minutes. Harolene has continued weight training two to three days per week, primarily sticking to upper body movements and lighter weights for 15 to 20 repetitions. Her running and weight workouts are supplemented by basic calisthenics every evening, stationary bike riding at medium intensity for 20–30 minutes 3 times per week, occasional half-hour swims, and 15–20 mile bike rides about twice per month on the weekend after a race. And, oh yes, Harolene runs as many as several races a month, racing almost every weekend.

In a few short years of intensive training, Harolene's talent and dedication have resulted in a string of impressive American age records.

Of course, readers can clearly see that between 43 and 44, Harolene showed some impressive improvement.

Over the years, Harolene has considerably modified her diet so that the word *stringent* seems a most appropriate descrip-

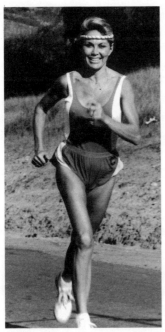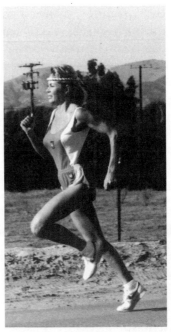

Harolene trains very hard, but as these pictures show, she enjoys her training and has great form.

tion. The bulk of her diet revolves around complex carbohydrates such as fruit, vegetables, rice, and beans. A good deal of her protein comes from yogurt and cottage cheese. She eats meat only about once a month. Because Harolene frequently runs in warm weather, she tries to drink eight glasses of water each day. Her basic diet is also supplemented by multivitamins, minerals, and calcium.

TABLE 13

Age 43:
    5K—17:42
    8K—29:17
    ½ marathon—1:24:33

Age 44:
    5K—17:30
    8K—29:03
    ½ marathon—1:20:32
    Marathon—2:47:33

Since Harolene was not a competitive runner in her 30s, it is difficult for her to assess changes in how she feels or performs that may be attributable to aging. Harolene does have a recurrent hamstring problem, and she has found that it is necessary to stretch both before and after she runs. Even when the hamstring problem flares up, she won't skip a workout. Instead, Harolene will usually do the same workout as scheduled, but at a slower pace. It is safe to say that at 45, Harolene looks, feels, and indeed is fitter and stronger than in her 30s. And, despite her very rigorous training schedule, Harolene has remained relatively injury-free.

Goals, Supports, Personal Processes

In January 1987, Harolene achieved a major goal that many runners aim for, but few reach. At the age of 44, Harolene qualified for the 1988 Olympic Trials by running a 2:47:00 time in the Phoenix Marathon. Incidentally, she also won the race.

Rather than seeing that achievement as the peak point in her career, Harolene, as we saw in the introduction, still feels that she can improve. Her second major goal is to improve her 10K time from about 36 minutes to 33 to 34 minutes. Thus, while many runners her age are content to maintain their times or accept some dropoff, Harolene is bent on improvement. And as the quote in the beginning of this portrait indicated, Harolene will be going after a bevy of age records throughout 1988.

To Harolene, training is usually satisfying and often enjoyable, but it is also serious business. She accepts the discomfort (and sometimes pain) of hard workouts, and pushes herself through them. Her husband Ron not only provides support and coaching, but also almost always is training right alongside Harolene. Ron plans Harolene's workouts and helps her monitor her efforts and recovery. In addition, many of Harolene's friends have taken an interest in all aspects of her training and success.

Harolene's success has also brought some well-deserved rewards, including prize money, trips, clothes, and watches. Most recently, she has been featured in national magazines, a

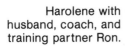

Harolene with husband, coach, and training partner Ron.

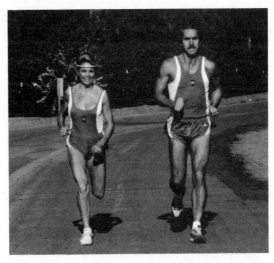

great sign of achievement for any athlete. Harolene has used the recent media attention as a way to make public commitments. For example, in a newspaper article Harolene was quoted as saying she planned on qualifying for the Olympic Trials and setting age records.

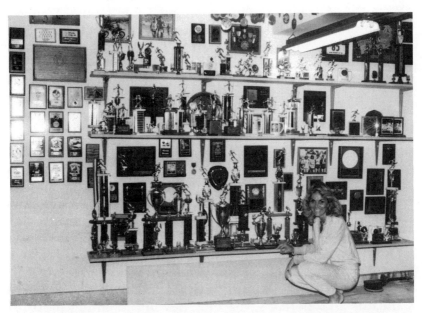

The trophies and awards Harolene has won in a few short years.

Harolene also really enjoys the company and the closeness of other runners. Their support keeps her very motivated, and Harolene will occasionally "brag" about recent wins to them to keep herself even more motivated.

Two important role models for Harolene are Priscilla Welch and Gabriele Anderson. These women are generally acknowledged to be the best masters runners in the world. They are highly visible on the international scene, yet open and accommodating to other runners. Harolene had interesting comments about the effects of these two athletes on her and what may be a final result of the modeling process:

> I really admire their accomplishments and wish that I could run as well as they do. I read about their workouts and sometimes try to put in as many miles as they do, but it's tough since I work full-time as a special education teacher. I believe, though, that if I ever really decided to get "super" serious about my running, I'd quit my job, get a coach, lose about five pounds, run a lot more miles and point for the big races. Then I might be able to come close to Priscilla and Gabriele.

Of course, Harolene is also becoming a role model. Younger women are amazed that a 45-year-old can run that fast, and middle-aged women are inspired by her good looks and athletic prowess. The attention and admiration of women across a wide age range keep Harolene highly motivated to train intensely and maintain her stature and self-esteem. However, Harolene is quick to add that: "I just like to compete and win, so a lot of my motivation flows from within myself." On the other hand, media attention and becoming a role model have some costs. For example, Harolene feels that she "needs to continuously run faster to maintain her image as a top masters runner," and she finds herself "constantly thinking about how I could improve my training schedules."

Harolene's personal standards—to be a top masters runner and record holder—are very high, and her success, as we have seen, has her thinking about even higher standards of excellence—world-class performances. Maintaining her personal standards and, perhaps, reaching beyond them has most recently entailed a closer monitoring of training and racing performance. Critical variables that she tracks mostly relate to speed, for example, how good or bad she feels when running intervals, or splits during races. This tracking not only provides a barometer of where Harolene is at a given point, but also tells her what her likely times will be in upcoming races and what she must do to improve upon them.

Harolene attaches considerable meaning to meeting or not meeting her personal standards. Meeting goals and standards makes Harolene feel elated and even more motivated to train harder to reach her next series of goals. She is likely to reward success with some food treat. Failure to meet goals and standards leads to depression and sometimes to following an even more rigid diet or training regime. However, Harolene's depression quickly subsides, to be replaced by a resolve not to give up and specific plans that will improve her times. Thus, with Harolene, her responses to victory or defeat seem very adaptive. In both instances, motivation is heightened and she will often train harder, but in a well-planned way.

While still searching for a more optimal training schedule and environment, Harolene remains very confident in her own abilities. This confidence, as we have seen, is not so much in her natural athletic abilities, but in her willingness to work exceedingly hard to reach her goals. "I feel that I can always achieve my goals if I put in enough time and effort," says Harolene. "I truly believe in myself."

While Harolene is beginning to reap some of the social and material rewards that accrue to top athletes, as we have seen, these rewards have commensurate costs. For Harolene, these costs have included over five years of hard training and rigorous nutritional practices. While the supports and rewards are important, most of her motivation comes from her high standards, love of competition and winning, and just plain desire for self-improvement. Or, as Harolene states:

As long as I'm able to run, I'll want to always be competitive and improve my times . . . so as long as I'm healthy, I'll be motivated to train intensely and compete in races.

HARRIET WEVER

In a note that accompanied Harriet Wever's completed and extremely detailed questionnaire, she said:

> I'm glad you asked me to participate. Because there are so few women my age on the running scene, I haven't found a role model, but it might just be that I can be a role model for women approaching the 60s. What an exciting thought!

Indeed, Harriet Wever not only can be a role model for the older runner, but a real inspiration for any middle-aged athlete or would-be athlete. For all of us, her example shows that at virtually any age and with almost any background, a person can reap the joys and benefits of a program of self-improvement.

Background

Harriet Wever was born in November 1921. At 67, Harriet is the oldest athlete featured in this book. She has been married to Dick for 40 years and is the mother of three daughters: Hila, 38; Kari, 36; and Nancy, 33; and grandmother to Derek, 8; Bree, 3; and Andrew, 3. Harriet received her B.A. degree from Michigan State University. When Hila started college in 1968, she went to work at MSU. Harriet has worked in various secretarial capacities at the university.

Harriet was never a physically active person. Her main recreational pursuits were reading and playing bridge. But when she started running, she had two things in her favor—she had never had a weight problem, and she had never smoked. It wasn't until she went along with her husband and daughter Kari to a road race that she decided to give running a try. Harriet was surprised to see a middle-aged woman running with her family and it looked like fun. She realized that running was something "old ladies" could do.

At Kari's urging, Harriet began training in August 1978 for a local women's 10K race. A stress fracture precluded her entering the race, but she got through her injury and kept training.

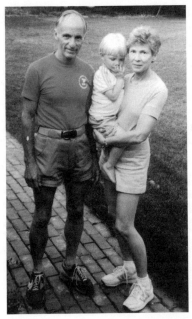

Harriet, husband Dick, and their grandson.

Harriet and her daughter Kari.

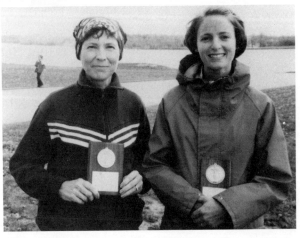

Her original goals in racing were to finish and not be last. Of course, Harriet has done much more than that as shown in Table 14, which lists the long string of single age records that she holds or has held.

The table is revealing in two ways. First, it shows a high level of consistency across a seven-year period. Second, and per-

Table 14

Age	Records
59	10 miles (1:26:30)
	½ marathon (1:56:42)
60	8K (37:58)
	10 miles (1:22:55)
	½ marathon (1:49:08)
61	5K (23:59)
	8K (39:17)
62	25K (2:16:06)
63	5K (24:16)
64	5K (24:00)
	8K (38:55)
	10K (48:38)
	25K (2:18:30)
	10 miles (1:22:23)
	½ marathon (1:47:44)
	15K (1:15:19)
65	5K (23:55)
	10 miles (1:20:22)

haps astonishing to some readers, is that Harriet's times in the longer races (10 miles and the half-marathon) have improved throughout her 60s! An examination of Harriet's goals, training, and motivational processes gives valuable information about developing and maintaining excellence.

Motivation: External Processes

Harriet decidedly does not fit the image of an older noncompetitive runner who ventures out for leisurely jaunts. Quite the contrary—Harriet is competitive and goal-oriented. As she states:

> My first goal was to FINISH and not be LAST. Then my goal became to improve my times, and to win the age category in which I was entered. That was sometimes 40 and up, and I often was first in that class. When I discovered national record keeping existed, my goal became to run as fast as, or faster than, the

existing record—a whole new challenge! Running a variety of distances has also been a part of my goals.

Later Harriet said:

> Racing keeps me running. The exhilaration of finishing a hard effort, the feelings of "well done" or "you can do better" make the training worthwhile. That means setting goals, monitoring performance, and competing.

Thus, competing and establishing new age records are Harriet's major goals as a runner. Harriet readily acknowledges that she needs upcoming competitions to keep her training intensity. To go through a tough workout, Harriet feels she must be aiming for a competition and have a specific program and workout plan. At times, she has found it is also necessary to gather some confidence and inspiration from looking at pictures of her winning past races. And, she will occasionally use positive self-statements to get through a difficult workout. For example, Harriet will keep telling herself:

> I am a good runner. I can easily run 8:00 miles. My legs feel good. My breathing is easy. I have plenty of power to continue this pace for 6 miles.

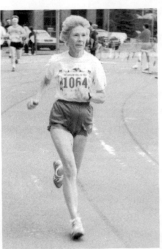

Picking up the pace at the end of a race.

Not surprisingly, Harriet has a specific plan for each race. She usually has planned ahead the overall time she wants to run, her splits, and times for each mile.

Harriet generally does her training runs alone, but occasionally she runs with Dick or Kari. Dick, Harriet feels, is most responsible for her start and career in running. "He supports me, encourages me, and brags about me . . . He keeps me on the road when I'd rather sit than run." Harriet loves sharing all the details of racing, training, encouragement, discouragement, and pride of racing with Kari. "We share many things, but this is special."

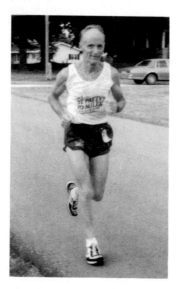

Harriet's favorite masters runner.

Hila and Nancy live 600 miles away, so even though Hila runs for fitness and does a few races each year, they haven't the same close sharing. Both daughters are interested and proud, however. Hila once introduced Harriet to a running friend of hers with, "This is Harriet Wever, my famous mother," much to Harriet's amusement.

However, unlike other national champions, Harriet does not have a coach, does not belong to an athletic organization, has rarely been featured in magazines or newspapers, and has received no real financial returns from her victories. Harriet does not feel that she would like a lot of publicity. In a number of ways, she feels it would be a burden; however, awards ceremonies at races and seeing her records in print remain important to Harriet. As she said:

> I suppose it reaffirms what I have accomplished. Being a wife, mother, a secretary, a grandmother, has limited applause. Maybe I need the affirmation of excellence on a larger scale.

Thus, again, prime motivators for Harriet are racing well and setting goals. Two other techniques enhance these motivators. Harriet keeps a very detailed log of her training runs and races. She uses her log to analyze her performance, to find out what she did right or wrong, to seek ways to improve, and to reach new goals. Harriet also feels a keen commitment to appear in her best possible condition when she is invited to a race. And, occasionally, she will make a public projection of her race time, a practice that Harriet has found to be very motivational. While Harriet is usually successful, failure to meet expectations results in some embarrassment and a great desire to do better at the next race.

The reactions of people of different ages to Harriet's prowess have also been interesting. Harriet noted that most younger people have been very enthusiastic about her running. Often, young people will approach her and say, "I think you're fantastic. I wish my mother would run." Harriet finds such comments delightful. She is glad the younger people do not feel an age barrier and can talk with her as they would a peer.

Same-aged people have mostly expressed approval and admiration for her running, although Harriet said that there are some who will persist in telling her why running is not good for people. Such comments do not bother her. "They can't change the fact that for me running is exciting and fulfilling, a great way to stay young in spirit."

Personal Motivational Processes

Harriet has very high personal standards that she sets for herself, yet, at the same time, she has learned to keep running and competition in perspective. Her standard is to be the best in her age category and to meet that standard by being out on the road training every day. Harriet says that matching or exceeding her personal standards is "one of the most important parts of my life." She added that:

> Running is an important part of my life. It requires stretching, reaching out; it challenges and motivates at an age when it seems more normal to sit back and relax. But I have to keep my perspective—running is only a sport. It is not the main business of my life. It can easily become all-consuming. In that context, matching or exceeding my personal standards is very important, but not the most important part of my life.

Another way Harriet keeps things in perspective is to realize that while on the one hand she is the pace setter in her age category, her personal level of excellence is only outstanding in comparison to same- and similar-aged women. In addition, she sees that some of the women moving up in age categories will be capable of breaking her records, just as she was able to break the records of women competing before her. However, Harriet feels that "It's exciting to be part of that process."

Harriet's use of a detailed training log was mentioned before as one way she constantly analyzes her performances. However, Harriet feels the best measure of her condition at any point is her performance in a race. Therefore, when training for a major race, Harriet will enter a few minor races to assess her condition and how her training is progressing. In her training and racing, Harriet focuses on her speed and endurance. She will, for example, check her time for each mile in a 10K race and see how she holds her pace throughout a race.

Harriet's moods often are related to how well she is meeting her standards. A good race and a good time will make Harriet feel elated, excited, and talkative. "I love everybody and am pretty pleased with myself." Harriet, of course, has known disappointment and discouragement from subpar performances. She tries not to dwell on the disappointment and does not let poorer performances affect how she acts toward others.

Harriet has a good deal of confidence in her training program (see below) because it has allowed her to perform well at a number of distances. Lately she has been thinking about adding some speed work but is not sure if she could handle more intensive training. Harriet did have a time, in 1984, when she went through two injuries that greatly limited her training for seven months. It was a time of major disappointment, and she questioned whether she could ever run and compete well again. With encouragement from Dick and Kari, she persisted and came back to have a very successful year in 1986. Based on this experience and her record of achievement, Harriet has considerable confidence in her abilities. As we saw before, at longer distances, Harriet is still improving. In Harriet's own words:

> The successes I've had so far have indicated that each year I'm running a little better. I believe I can still improve. I think I have more ability than I've demonstrated so far. Isn't that what keeps us coming back for more?

Training, Aging, and the Future

Harriet does most of her training on the country roads around her home. When she is not working, she tries to run in the mid-morning. When she is working, her schedule becomes more complicated. However, Harriet will always get her training in even if it means running in the late evening. Since Dick is also a runner, sticking to her training schedule has not caused many problems.

Harriet has a base program where she runs between 25 and 30 miles per week following a simple schedule such as: Monday-3 miles; Tuesday-5 miles; Wednesday-7 miles; Thursday-3 miles; Friday-5 miles; Saturday-8 to 10 miles; Sunday-off. As noted before, Harriet does not do any speed work, although she is contemplating that for the future. The minor races she runs in her buildups to major races serve as speed work. She is careful with these all-out efforts because she has always had some recovery problems from them. And, the primary goal of her program is to develop endurance with lower-intensity training. Harriet does not do hill training since the area where she lives is flat.

Harriet and Dick follow a normal, not extreme, runner's diet. They emphasize complex carbohydrates, but do eat meat and have desserts in moderation.

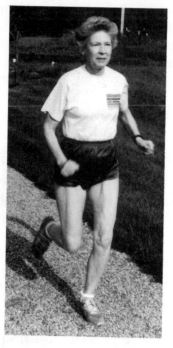

A relaxed training run.

Overall, Harriet recognizes a number of physical changes that appear attributable to aging. These changes include joint stiffness, diminished eyesight, some hearing loss, and difficulty in adjusting to temperature extremes. None of the changes has presented major problems. However, Harriet can foresee a time when she will have to run later in the day when she is less stiff and start out slower. She may also have to be more careful on the roads and avoid racing in hot, humid weather.

Harriet's knees are also sensitive and she has had left foot and toe problems. She uses a metatarsal pad in her running shoes, tries to stick to blacktop surfaces, and does not race beyond the 25K distance. However, lest readers conclude that Harriet is starting an inevitable slide, she reports that in the last few years, she has become decidedly stronger. She notices better muscle tone in her legs, more lower body development in general, and a greater ability to hold a pace in her races. She is also finding that she has less problems now with upper respiratory infections and sore muscles after races.

Indeed, it can be predicted that some of Harriet's best years are ahead of her and that she will serve as role model for many present and future athletes. Is there a time ahead when Harriet's motivation for training and competing will wane and her injuries and aging will catch up to her? Harriet says:

> I don't foresee any physical problems that will keep me from running. I expect to keep on running and racing well into my 80s.

FRANK ZANE

It would be easy to fill any number of pages describing Frank Zane's career in bodybuilding. After all, Frank has won the Mr. America, Mr. World, Mr. Universe (three times), and Mr. Olympia (three times) titles. Frank represented an entirely different, albeit short-lived, trend in bodybuilding that can be called the "Apollo" era. He is statuesque, probably the most perfectly proportional bodybuilder in history. These are qualities that appear largely lost in today's emphasis on pure muscle mass and definition.

Optimistically, it may be said that Frank was always ahead of his time and that in a few years trends in bodybuilding will catch up to where Frank was 10 to 15 years ago. Frank is still on the cutting edge of the sport. It makes sense, then, to briefly describe Frank's earlier years and take more space to describe where Frank is now in his mid-40s and how his life is evolving.

Earlier Years

Frank was born in June 1942, in Kingston, Pennsylvania. As a child and early adolescent, Frank was very studious and reflective, shy, and a bit of a loner. Physically, he was unremarkable; indeed, he was quite thin and undeveloped. At the age of 14,

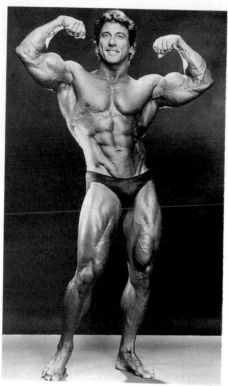

Frank epitomizes the "Apollo" tradition in bodybuilding.

Frank made an important discovery. In searching for ways to build up his body for high school sports, he discovered weight training. However, these were the 1950s, and Frank was discouraged from continuing weight training by his parents, coaches, and peers. As soon as he started lifting weights, though, Frank knew he was on to something. Very quickly, Frank perceived that he had a special, unique relationship with the weights. Not only did he enjoy the feeling of training, but within weeks of starting, he was able to see muscular changes.

Again, almost by accident, by looking through some bodybuilding magazines, Frank discovered that there were actually competitions. At the age of 18, Frank entered his first contest. He placed third in the teenage Mr. America contest. Frank readily admits that from that point on he was tremendously motivated by winning contests, titles, and trophies. He particularly liked the attention, recognition, and praise he was receiving.

Very early on, Frank also displayed a highly systematic and well-planned approach. He set specific contests and titles to achieve as goals. These contests represented a succession of hard but reachable goals, one of the primary motivation strategies discussed at length in Chapter 2.

By the time he was 22, Frank had received his bachelors degree in secondary education from Wilkes College. For 13 years, Frank taught in a number of public schools on the East Coast, Florida, and California. He found teaching to be enjoyable, and during the 1960s and 1970s ample positions meant that considerable mobility was possible. This allowed Frank to experiment with various locations and training environments. In addition, the school year schedule fit nicely with the competitive bodybuilding season.

In this respect, Frank was one of the first bodybuilders to systematically cycle his training phases, a practice he still follows today. Obviously, this is also consistent with the periodization model described in Chapter 3. Fall until early winter is usually a period of low-key training and general conditioning. From early winter to early spring, training intensity and volume pick up a bit. Both intensity, volume, and sometimes frequency are increased even more from early spring to early summer. During the summer, all training variables are at their maximum level, and intensity may even be turned up another notch by decreasing the rest time between sets.

Frank's peaking phase coincided with his summer vacations. Thus, while he was training very intensely, he was also able to take more time for recovery purposes, a point emphasized in Chapter 3.

Mid-30s to Present

By the time Frank was in his 30s, bodybuilding was starting to become much more popular. It was apparent that he could make a good deal of money at the sport. Some of Frank's business interests have included mail-order training courses, a number of excellently put together books that sell well, mail-order amino acid and vitamin supplements, and training semi-nars. However, by far his most extensive and exciting business venture has been the creation and operation of "Zane Haven," to be described later.

What is also so intriguing (and encouraging) about Frank is that during his early middle years he has kept evolving person-ally and professionally. Frank feels that today he is more out-going, relaxed, and confident than he was in his 30s. He is currently working on an advanced degree in psychology so that he will understand the psychological underpinnings of training and other health-related behaviors and be able to use them effectively. His knowledge of psychology is very broad. He is well-versed in behavioral psychology, psychoanalysis, and a life-span developmental perspective, and he is currently doing research in unconscious learning. He may well become one of the few people to be able to successfully integrate diverse positions and move beyond his current eclectic stance.

Frank readily admits that he is very motivated to become even more successful financially. Yet at the same time, he in-trinsically likes studying, gaining knowledge, and as we will see, being able to convey that knowledge to others.

Frank still adheres to a phase or training cycle system. He trains about 4 to 12 hours per week, weights and aerobics included. He no longer uses maximum weights, reasoning that perfectly executed repetitions with moderate weight, with an emphasis on the negative part of the movement, are particu-larly beneficial. His workouts are very fast-paced; he quickly moves from exercise to exercise.

Frank has also reduced his body weight. His highest compet-itive weight was about 200. Now he weighs about 170–175, the same weight he was in high school. To Frank, this is almost like a second adolescence! More to the point, though, Frank's ad-vice for all masters athletes is to get as lean as possible. There is no reason in the middle years to be walking around with any excess bulk.

Four to 12 hours of training per week is considerably less time than many masters athletes spend. Frank also spends about 30 minutes per day in a deeply relaxed state by listening to his unique mental power psycho-acoustical tapes in a dry flotation environment. Frank's "Mental Power Program" combines advanced audio and psychological technology and is structured for learning on both the conscious and unconscious levels. Frank feels that this contrasting combination of exercise and relaxation is more beneficial in the long run from a health and fitness perspective. Recent studies support his opinion. For example, it is doubtful that any amount of exercise can offset the detrimental effects on health of chronic distress.

Frank has always emphasized the duality of mind and body in fitness, high-level training, and competition. He was exploring the use of visualization techniques long before their use became more commonplace. Yet another example is his long-term systematic study of his own dreams. By recording his dreams and studying themes and patterns, Frank indicated that he can often work out solutions to future business, personal, or athletic problems.

Since Frank has taught math and science, it is not surprising that he uses this knowledge to quantify some of the interrelationships between diverse variables that must work in concert if high-level goals are to be reached. One interesting equation was developed during his competition days:

Goal (winning the contest) = Exercise × Attitude × Relaxation × Nutrition.

Not by coincidence, the first letters of the variables spell EARN. What is important about the formula as a heuristic (an informative set of guidelines) is the notion that the variables are in a multiplicative relationship. This means that even if a person were effectively operating at 90 percent for each variable, the sum total would be about 66 percent. Thus, a person would be far off their optimal performance level. Optimal performance requires that all essential inputs themselves be optimized.

Clearly, such heuristics can be applied to other diverse aspects of a person's life, such as family life and career success. One of Frank's future contributions may be to combine his background in mathematics with psychology and attempt to quantify important inputs and their respective weights and interrelationships to health. The use of computers and modern statistics makes such an endeavor more than a mere possibility.

Zane Haven

All of Frank's diverse interests appear to have come together in the development and operation of Zane Haven with his wife Christine. Remember that analyses of motivation should start with the environment. When the environment is not conducive to performing particular behaviors, only extraordinary personal initiative can overcome barriers to performance. Rather than constantly calling on extraordinary initiative, it makes much more sense to optimize the environment.

In Zane Haven, Frank has created the optimal environment for all his different interests. Located in Palm Springs, California, Zane Haven is a full-scale vacation resort for men and women at any level who want to learn more about and get a state-of-the-art, hands-on approach to health, fitness, and

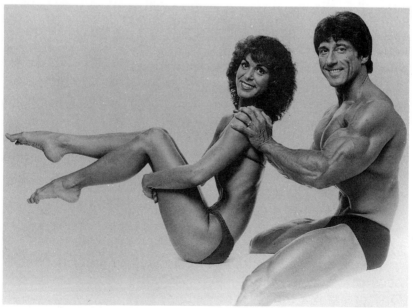

Frank and wife Christine—Is this middle age?

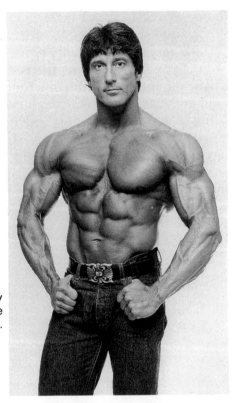

A picture that quickly shows why many still consider Frank the greatest bodybuilder.

bodybuilding. Frank and Christine work closely with small groups over a five-day period. This means there is not only instruction, but actual training sessions with them. Frank likens these short but intensive stays to effective, brief cognitive-behavioral psychotherapy.

These days, in fact, Frank does much of his training with his guests, a practice that he find keeps him highly motivated. Frank, after all, is the role model. In many ways Zane Haven is an extension of Frank and Christine's teaching careers, but now they teach small groups in their own setting. Zane Haven also is a place where Frank and Christine can experiment with new training, relaxation, and nutrition ideas.

Zane Haven has been a financial success. But Frank and Christine have not overemphasized the financial aspects of Zane Haven. Groups are kept small, and there may be only about 150 visitors a year. That means that since its opening, there have been about 1,000 people who have benefitted from this unique setting.

Frank said his personality type, as shown through the Myer-Briggs Type Indicator, fits the prototype of a scientist—an introverted, intuitive, thinking, judging type. Perhaps in Frank's younger years the scientist in him primarily focused on formulating relationships among bodybuilding variables. His middle years find him on the cutting edge of bodybuilding psychology. His ability to keep growing and evolving in his middle years, virtually following a renaissance ideal, can serve as a model for many of us.

6
Key Psychological and Training Elements of Masters Athletes: Analysis and Integration of the Portraits

Before I summarize the 17 portraits of masters athletes, let me be forthright at the outset and expand on some of the qualifying points noted in the introduction to the portraits. When you ask individuals particular questions in particular ways, it should not be surprising that you end up with particular responses. The way you frame inquiries plays a large hand in determining what you get; "Seek and you shall find."

The questionnaire and interviews closely revolved around the psychological systems framework presented in Chapter 2. Therefore, the data obtained fits into different parts of the framework. Perhaps if I had been an old dyed-in-the-wool psychoanalyst, I would have asked these athletes about their early toilet training and come up with some supportive findings!

That caveat being issued, it must be said that *it is compelling how closely the data presented in the portraits fit the psychological framework*. In the portraits, we see the rich interplay of cognitive, affective, behavioral, and environmental domains. The athletes have much in common in terms of these interplays, but they also demonstrate some unique aspects. Interestingly, there were no apparent differences in motivational strategies between men and women athletes. Indeed, the only apparent difference was in training. By and large, the men had been training for more years than the women—which probably says more about recent sociocultural changes than differences between the sexes.

While the framework for this book emphasizes interactions, it is first easier to look at important psychological elements one by one. Later, some of the commonalities and unique aspects of training and aging will be highlighted.

One other caveat must also be noted. In Chapter 2, we made a distinction between stages of behavior change—acquisition, generality, and sustained. Clearly, even those master athletes portrayed in this book who started their athletic activities in their 30s now are in the sustained stage.

The commonalities between the athletes, as well as each individual's uniqueness, teaches us a great deal about motivation and behavior. However, the novice athlete may want to reread and think about some of the change processes in the acquisition and generality stages discussed in Chapters 2 and 4. For example, the masters athletes portrayed in this book generally train alone and do not use ostensive incentives to keep them motivated. Beginners may need incentives and social supports to pursue rigorous training (Chapter 4).

PSYCHOLOGICAL ELEMENTS

Goal-Setting

There is one element that clearly runs through virtually every portrait to an extent that even surprised me. These individuals, some at early ages, some not until their middle years, learned the great value of *setting goals*. Often, these athletes set a series of hard but reachable goals (e.g., Al Oerter, Frank Zane), or set a long-term goal and then backtrack to the present and set up specific short-term goals (e.g., Bill Pearl). Many of the athletes were able to also adopt a long-term perspective on training and competing. For example, Harolene Walters is looking forward to record-setting years for the next decade;

Lucille Griffin realized in her middle 30s that it would probably take her 25 to 30 years to reach the top; Harriet Wever wants to be still running in her 80s.

Overall, the athletes followed an almost textbook process in goal-setting that sets them apart from most people. As some of the athletes pointed out to me, many people they encountered had no particular goals in any avenue of life.

The athletes are most adept at picking challenging, hard, but for them reachable goals (e.g., Harolene Walters), a type of goal-setting strategy that is most motivating. Once goals were picked, the athletes all had great ability to channel their efforts toward reaching their goals. In a word, they were able to maintain a real focus, to constantly "keep their eye on the ball." Of course, the ability to keep a focus is greatly enhanced, as we will shortly see, by arranging a supportive environment, choosing the right spots (i.e., the right goals, activities, and competitions), and having a history of success. Successes in meeting initial goals raise self-efficacy beliefs so that more challenging goals are pursued. Or, as Clarence Bass stated more simply and succinctly, "Success breeds success."

What is particularly refreshing is that as some of the athletes are getting older, they have learned to "not take themselves so seriously" (e.g., Clarence Bass again), to not be quite as driven as they were before. Even with (or perhaps because of) this more relaxed perspective, these athletes are still consistently achieving in sports and other parts of their lives.

For many of the athletes, winning competitions and setting records remain as major, highly motivating goals. This was true for the younger ageless athletes (e.g., Barry Brown, Barbara Filutze, Harolene Walters) and the older athletes (e.g., John Hosner, Harriet Wever). Other athletes, such as Al Oerter ("being there") and Joe Germana ("authentic involvement"), are learning that the activity and participation themselves are their own rewards. And, perhaps, John Gregg's "90 percent rule" (see p. 150) may be helpful to some overachieving and tightly wired masters athletes, while Frank Zane's "renaissance man" may become an interesting model for more single-focused individuals.

Environmental Design

As we discussed at length in Chapter 2, probably the best starting point for an analysis of motivation is an analysis of the environment. All too often psychological studies of individuals seem to forget that behavior is transacted in environments that can help or hinder an individual's best efforts. The athletes featured in this book all understand the importance of a supportive environment in their pursuit of excellence.

For many of the athletes, their daily schedule revolves around training. This does not mean that they do nothing else—hardly the case at all—but that getting in training is a top priority each day. Scheduling may mean following a meticulous hourly plan (e.g., Lynne Pirie), or simply being sure that a major workout occurs early in the day. This means that a number of the athletes train very early in the day (e.g., Bill Pearl at 3:30 A.M. and Tracy Smith at 5:30 A.M). There are exceptions to this rule. Some of the athletes train later in the day (e.g., Harolene Walters) or do not always have a fixed training time (e.g., John Gregg). However, regardless of the exact schedule, training time is carefully set aside virtually every day.

It must be acknowledged that most of the athletes are in jobs or careers with more flexible work schedules (e.g., Joe Germana) or in some cases work part-time (e.g., Barbara Filutze, Al Oerter, Harriet Wever). However, others are in incredibly demanding positions and careers, although their schedules can be flexible. For example, Clarence Bass is the sole practitioner in a busy law practice, John Hosner is the Dean of the Forestry and Wildlife School at Virginia Tech, Barry Brown heads his investment and consulting firm, Todd Scully is a coach and businessman, Harolene Walters is a special education teacher, and Lynne Pirie is in constant demand in her medical practice. Planning and scheduling for these individuals is extremely important. Only two individuals (Tracy Smith and Bobbi Rothman) can be considered full-time athletes.

Very often, the athletes have given much thought to the actual training environment. Clarence Bass and Bill Pearl have their own superbly equipped personal gyms. Barry Brown and

Al Oerter spend the warm months in the North and the winters in Florida. Harolene Walters can do great workouts on bike paths near her home. Lynne Pirie's training facilities are part of the health institute where she works. Bobbi Rothman and her husband retired early from their teaching careers so that Bobbi could train full-time in Florida. And, going one step further, Frank Zane, with Zane Haven, has created a total therapeutic and motivational environment for himself and his wife.

However, some of the other athletes have what must be considered only adequate facilities or surroundings that they have made work for them. Al Oerter only needs a high school throwing area, a bare-bones heavy gym, and an exercise bike. Todd Scully trains on the various roadways around Virginia Tech. Harriet Wever sticks to roads around her home. Tracy Smith has been able to make the rich countryside in California work to his benefit for relaxing mountain runs, and Barbara Filutze has even gained something from running through the Pennsylvania winters. In Barbara's case, the winter has provided a reprieve from the tough paces she runs in more benign seasons and a time to plan the coming year's goals on training runs with her husband. Thus, each athlete has tried to maximize their training environment in some way.

It is also interesting to assess what the training environments of these athletes do *not* include. Except for occasional training partners, most of the athletes train alone (or with a spouse). Bill Pearl, Frank Zane, and Bobbi Rothman are exceptions. A few of the athletes, such as Tracy Smith, have found that they do need training partners for their very hard workouts. It is also true that the portraits do not include athletes from team sports. Therefore, it is not surprising that the general image from the portraits is of a solitary athlete.

Except for advice and other occasional interactions with coaches, most of the athletes are self-coached. They do not have another person constantly pushing them. Again, a caveat is that these are veteran athletes with long years of experience. In the beginning, many of the athletes (e.g., Bill Pearl, Lynne Pirie, and Tracy Smith) could point to an inspirational coach.

As Al Oerter noted, he is not surrounded by an entourage.

That applies to all the athletes portrayed in this book. Agents, training partners, handlers, helpers, groupies, and others are nowhere to be seen. In fact, what was heartening was how open and accessible the athletes are (see Chapter 1).

This is partly the case because, with a few exceptions, these individuals have not become wealthy or well-known through their athletic prowess. In fact, a few world and national record holders are hardly known as athletes in their own communities. At a minimum, the portraits of these athletes tell us that often the benefits—and the trappings—of celebrity status are not necessary to become and continue to be a top athlete.

Self-Standards and Other Cognitive and Affective Processes

Coupled with their goal-setting strategies are the very high self-standards each athlete has. Of course, given their status and ability, it follows that their self-standards would be very high. Standards sometimes include winning every race or competition and, in one case, that of Barry Brown, it means changing the terrain to "completely redefine what a 40-year-old is capable of." Most generally, all the athletes have as their self-standard to "be the best they could be in their sport," "do the best they could do in each competition," and, some added, to "be the best human being possible."

Also, almost without exception, each athlete has great confidence (high self-efficacy) in their ability to perform based on their many successes over the years. Interestingly, self-efficacy beliefs often are based more on performance and psychological attributes such as perseverance and drive than on a sense of being genetically gifted. Good illustrations of this point are found in the portraits of Barry Brown, Bobbi Rothman, and Todd Scully.

Outcome expectancies, "confidence in the program," are also usually very high. As we will discuss, these athletes, often through trial and error, have developed a training program that worked for them. A number had, however, gone through periods of doubt in their ability and regime. Doubt often led to experimentation with new methods, and often a return to their own tried-and-true method.

Close self-observation of performance is a self-regulatory process all the athletes follow. Not every athlete used a training log for this purpose. Some used rudimentary training logs, while others (e.g., Bobbi Rothman) developed detailed logs that simultaneously tracked a number of physical and psychological processes. Whatever the method, the athletes are able to closely monitor several processes before, during, and after training sessions and competitions and make both midcourse corrections and later adaptations.

For example, Frank Zane could channel his condition to such an extent that he could reach a peak at literally an exact moment. Bobbi Rothman makes changes before and during workouts based on her perceptions of recovery. Lucille Griffin always monitors her swimming form and knows which form gives her the best performance with the least risk of injury.

These hyper-vigilant and sensitive self-observation processes are a good example of "self-biofeedback." Many of the athletes I know constantly engage in these processes while most of the nonathletes I know do not. The self-observation, feedback, and behavior change loop appears to be an important part of athletic success and remaining healthy despite the stresses athletes place upon themselves. It is likely that the general population can gain a healthy advantage by learning these processes.

In another realm, considerable affect is attached to exceeding, meeting, or not meeting training and competition standards and goals. In a word, athletics is a top priority and provides structure and meaning to the lives of these individuals (although all the athletes pointed out that training and competition is *not* their number one priority). Not surprisingly, depression and elation, "the agony and ecstasy," comes with athletic performance.

These masters athletes have learned to enjoy moments of triumph and goal attainment. However, they realize that, on the one hand, you're only as good as your last competition, while on the other hand, a lot of the enjoyment and satisfaction is in the doing and striving. So, it's on to the next workout and goal. In fact, John Gregg and others described this elation from workouts and competitions as a main element in their longevity. Harriet Wever talked about always wanting to see if she could improve just a bit more.

Doubt and depression are also part of the process. Perhaps because of their age and backgrounds in general, these masters athletes did not dwell on their failures. Yes, subpar performances do bring on some depression; however, depression is often a stimulus for constructive self-analysis (e.g., of training and competition preparation) and change. These athletes keep both their triumphs and defeats in perspective.

What about the role of "higher order beliefs" in these athletes' motivation and performance? Only two individuals, Tracy Smith and Beverly Crown, can be considered motivated by religious or religious-like feelings and beliefs. Tracy Smith has his profound feelings of virtually "running for God." Beverly Crown has equally intense feelings that training helps her literally maintain herself in the struggle of life.

As noted above, most of these athletes have not received public accolades for either their perseverance or triumphs. Often, the only real encouragement and positive reinforcement may come from a spouse or a few other masters athletes. Occasionally, these masters athletes may create a motivational environment for themselves, if for only a moment, by the use of a public commitment strategy (e.g., announcing they will win the next race) or by giving newspapers interviews and stories about themselves. But these are not prime motivators. At the core, these athletes are not in it, as younger athletes might be, for social status and peer praise. Indeed, the responses from same-aged peers is often mixed—admiration, wonder, and derision.

In the end, we have the persevering ageless athlete, often striving alone, but with great satisfaction, to meet lofty goals and standards through careful self-observation and feedback, planning, and environmental design.

AGING AND TRAINING

Aging

There is a 30-year age span, 38 to 68, for the masters athletes featured in this book. Thus, the athletes range from very early to very late middle age, a period when substantial aging and physical decline is supposed to take place.

At least as far as performance, long-time younger ageless athletes, along with Clarence Bass and Al Oerter (50 and 51, respectively) generally do not show any substantial performance decrements. This is particularly the case for strength athletes; if anything, they report that they are stronger than ever before. It appears to be less the case for aerobic athletes. There are exceptions, however, in all possible categories.

John Gregg reported, for example, that his performance decreases have been in part attributable to his training schedule and some concomitant family problems in the recent past. Todd Scully reports he is faster at 40 than in his 20s and 30s. Tracy Smith is approaching his performances of 20 years ago. John Hosner at 62 and Lucille Griffin at 50 are making PRs. Today, Bill Pearl, in his late 50s, looks more muscular and defined (if that's possible) than in his Mr. Universe days. And the late starters, Bobbi Rothman, Barbara Filutze, Harolene Walters, and Joe Germana, keep improving in their 40s.

Of course, all the athletes today are training "smarter" than they did years ago. Smarter includes the type of training schedule, to be discussed at length shortly, nutritional practices, and adjunct training activities. Most of the athletes have become much more conscious of and conscientious about nutrition. Their dietary practices are similar—low-fat, high-complex carbohydrates, moderate protein. This is exactly the kind of diet now recommended by the American Heart Association and the National Cancer Institute. The strength athletes emphasize more protein and dietary supplements (see Chapter 2), while typically the endurance athletes consume more calories.

Two common signs of aging noted by many of the athletes were stiffness, particularly in the mornings, and some noticeably slower recovery from hard workouts. Many of the athletes have added stretching to their training regimes and are more careful about the time interval between hard workouts.

Training

Although the training programs of the athletes seem to be

very different, there are some important commonalities. First and foremost is that all the athletes really *enjoy* their training. They have a fascination with improvement and derive a great deal of satisfaction from their efforts. The athletes have learned to construct their training schedules so that they look forward to training instead of dreading it.

For many readers, this point, so central to motivation and longevity, may seem obvious and not worth mentioning. In contrast, I feel it is a point to be made again and again. Athletes have it within their power to make their training challenging and enjoyable. This simple insight starts a "reverberating" and "upward spiralling" effect discussed and shown in Chapter 2.

This point doesn't seem to be recognized by many beginning athletes and fitness buffs and is not emphasized enough in various local, commercial, and national programs to promote health and fitness. Make a program interesting and enjoyable—if it isn't, change it! If the program is boring or too hard, do not be surprised that no one will follow it for very long.

A second commonality is that all the athletes, after experimentation, believe that their training program is the best one for them. Whether it is true or not that different individuals respond very differently to different training regimes (or whether there is a "best approach"—see Chapter 3) remains a conjecture. In the end, highly positive outcome expectancies (belief in the program) may be a most critical factor for success.

A third commonality is that most of the programs revolve around the concept of hard and easy days. No one is training hard every day of the week for a good reason—it doesn't work. Typically, athletes use two or three hard sessions per week and have two or three easier days between hard workouts. Strength athletes can put more hard days together when they use split routines, but by and large, these athletes train body parts once hard and once easy during a week. Bill Pearl appears to train hard every day, but actually Pearl's training emphasizes use of more moderate weights (see pp. 181 to 191).

A fourth commonality is that the hard workouts are, indeed,

very hard. Hard workouts are exemplified by Barry Brown's and Tracy Smith's (see pp. 114 to 123), Barbara Filutze's (see pp. 131 to 141), and Tracy Smith's (see pp. 216 to 225) athletes frequently prepare for such hard workouts by having easier days precede them and by using visualization strategies, also days before the big workout. The athlete visualizes successfully completing chunks of the workout.

A fifth commonality is that almost all the athletes use a kind of periodization approach. Their training tends to be seasonal in that certain parts of a year regularly feature very hard training, while other parts of the year consist of lower-intensity training. None of the athletes train hard every month of the year.

Except for Clarence Bass, no one appeared to closely follow the periodization model of Chapter 3. I believe, though, that many of the athletes do follow a periodization model in two ways. They have systematic buildups during a year for competitions, and by keen self-observations know when to push ahead or back off (e.g., see Bobbi Rothman, pp. 200 to 209). Thus the spirit, if not exact laws, of periodization is generally followed.

The aerobic athletes profiled here do not completely follow the suggestion in Chapter 3 that aerobic athletes adopt the effective tenets of strength programs, namely, relatively infrequent but intense sessions. As noted, the aerobic athletes in this book all tend to follow a hard-easy day system. However, often there did not appear to be a great deal of difference between hard and easy days (e.g., see John Hosner, pp. 163 to 172 and Harriet Wever, pp. 234 to 243). A real exception to this pattern is Tracy Smith. His training program (see pp. 216 to 225) most closely followed the principles discussed in Chapter 3.

The athletes differ the most in their volume of workload and duration of training. For example, in volume and duration, the training schedules of Bill Pearl versus Clarence Bass and Barry Brown versus Tracy Smith differ by a factor of about 2½ to 1. This is quite a bit of difference! Yet, as noted, there are actually commonalities between the programs and, for a variety of reasons, all the athletes felt their programs were the best for them.

Conclusions

What can be concluded on balance about aging, training, and performance? It must be conceded that only two of the athletes—Todd Scully and Al Oerter—consider themselves top national-level athletes in open competition. Clarence Bass, Beverly Crown, Bill Pearl, and Frank Zane—all bodybuilders—*may* be able to do terrifically well in open competition, but that is no longer their goal. Tracy Smith is approaching the performances of his youth, and Barry Brown is still a threat in some open races.

One supposition is that in sports where there are many variables within an athlete's control that contribute to peak performance, top competitive days may be greatly extended. For example, in bodybuilding (strength does not appear to decline much, if at all, in earlier middle age), a better training regime, nutritional practices, and weight control can lead a top masters athlete to look much better than 10 to 15 years previously. This may be the case even when recovery and flexibility are not quite what they were.

There is, however, an anomaly in masters bodybuilders' appearances. Often, their bodies will look the same as, or even better than, top competitors 20 years their junior. However, facially many may look their age or at least in the chronological ballpark (for an exception, see Beverly Crown's pictures on pp. 125 and 130). What the anomaly means may be revealed as top strength athletes continue to train intensely beyond middle age.

In aerobic sports similar compensations can be made, but to a lesser extent. In most cases, an aerobic masters athlete does not compete in open competition. And with a few exceptions (e.g., Barry Brown), aerobic athletes tend to look their age.

It is safe to say that much of the "inevitable physical decline" thought to "naturally" occur in the 40s and perhaps even 50s is not so inevitable. Yes, there are changes and even some loss, but a good deal of change may be compensated for by intelligent training and health practices.

In the end, we come back to the example of an interesting reciprocal relationship we started with in Chapter 2. If you think you will decline in your 40s and 50s, you will probably decrease your training intensity and perhaps not be as concerned or careful about training, nutrition, and rest. The result is reduced ability and performance, confirming your belief, and thus leading to further reductions in athletic behavior and so on—our "downward spiral" and a great example of a "self-fulfilling prophecy."

If, however, you believe that physical ability and performance will only decline minimally, almost imperceptibly, in your middle years, things will shape up quite differently. You are likely to continue to train hard, but intelligently and in a challenging and enjoyable way, closely monitor recovery and performance, and follow good nutritional and health practices. You may find yourself not only holding your own but actually improving in an exciting "upward spiral," another positive example of a self-fulfilling prophecy.

It may be a safe bet that a 48-year-old runner will not win the Boston, New York, Chicago, or Olympic marathons. But if you knew that some great runners of the past, now in their middle 40s, were in serious training, you may not want to bet against a 45-year-old accomplishing that feat. Of course, the great Priscilla Welch, just a shade short of 43, ran away from the field and won the 1987 New York Marathon!

And you'd best be careful not to bet against a 57-year-old winning an open Universe or Olympia title. Albert Beckles, at 57, placed tenth in the pinnacle of bodybuilding, the 1987 Mr. Olympia Contest!

7
What All This Means for You/ Postscript

One of the original objectives of this book—which was quickly discarded—was to review theories of aging as they related to athletics and performance. These theories include genetic theories of aging emphasizing a predetermined life span, theories of DNA breakdown, theories concerned with free radical exposure which disrupts DNA replication, and theories that focus more on the endocrine and immune systems. This work has been nicely reviewed in the book by Jan and Terry Todd noted in Chapter 1.

These theories are still in the early experimentation stage. It is unclear, except in the case of Roy Walford's theory which prescribes a low-calorie but maximally nutritious diet, what these theories can prescriptively offer us to increase longevity and the quality of life.

A psychological perspective is also informing us about aging. This perspective is providing some straightforward ideas, particularly about cognitive, affective, environmental (sociocultural), and behavioral aspects of aging.

The most dramatic changes concerning aging are occurring right before our eyes. As little as 10 to 15 years ago, the notion of middle-aged men and women training and competing at high levels would have seemed strange to scientists and the general public. Middle-aged athletes are changing our socio-cultural beliefs about what it means to be middle-aged. At the same time athletes, such as the ones featured in this book are providing explicit life-style and performance models. These models are inspiring countless individuals to try their hand at, or continue in, athletics. As more people emulate models and take up athletics, a profound evolution in beliefs and feelings on an individual and societal level about the capabilities of middle-aged people gains momentum. The success of each individual feeds back into the overall process.

At the same time, the greater acceptance of middle-aged athletes leads to more pathways for performance, including many new gyms and masters competitions. These factors are providing the impetus, social reinforcement, and social and physical settings that further enhance athletics for the middle-aged.

Thus, again, it is possible on a larger scale to see the reciprocity of environmental, behavioral, cognitive, and affective domains, as these many factors interact to create the middle-aged athlete. However, just as we have emphasized for individual examples in Chapters 2, 3, and 4, note how on a larger scale all these factors are interacting in a positive and highly synergistic way—again, our "upward spiralling" phenomenon. In a nutshell, the psychological framework of this book is useful for also examining sociocultural changes, and in this case, where the process will stop is uncertain. As the last chapter ended, for example, we were contemplating over-50-year-old athletes successfully competing in open events at the highest level.

If one main facet of aging has to do with function and performance, we can conclude that, in part, what was usually thought of as a natural accompaniment of aging in the middle years has much to do with disuse. The old adage of "use it or lose it" has a good deal of wisdom. In the function and performance sense, the day you stop exercising and training is the day you start to age. And for those who are still sedentary, the day you start exercising and training is the day you begin to become younger!

Since exercise and training are central to the discussion, it is important not only to review some of the main points emphasized in this book, but also to add a number of germane points.

EXERCISE AND TRAINING

The Right Activity

Many of the athletes featured in this book have pointed to their drive and perseverance, rather than genetic gifts, as the key attributes in their success. However, without exception, each athlete concurs that they are involved in a sport that ideally suits them temperamentally and genetically. Certain individuals are just better designed for running long distances, sprinting, swimming, bodybuilding, or weightlifting. This does not mean that you must restrict yourself to only those few select activities you can do well in. In fact, a few athletes, such as John Gregg, prefer to be involved in many types of activities and sports.

However, we know that a major aspect of motivation and longevity in sports has to do with the performance feedback you receive. The feedback, as we have seen, colors your affect, beliefs, and subsequent performances and feedback. For most individuals, the contrasting feedback between doing an activity well and with ease versus with mediocrity and injury, will have obvious short- and long-term impacts.

A simple personal example, which picks up from some of the discussion in Chapter 1, illustrates this point. I recounted how, in my 30s, I ran many miles including speedwork and overdistance but never really enjoyed running that much and never could run very well. In fact, putting together two or three 6:30 miles was usually a big accomplishment for me.

About the time when I wanted to cut down my running while continuing to do a lot of aerobics, I read about the Schwinn Air Dyne. The Air Dyne is a flywheel exercise bike that also has a synchronized push-pull arm motion. The harder you cycle and push and pull, the greater the resistance. The apparatus can give you a great whole-body aerobic workout without impact stress or overworking particular body parts.

After I read about the Air Dyne, I knew I had to try one. I wasn't disappointed. The first time I tried one in a store, I felt comfortable and was able to work at a high level. I bought the Air Dyne on the spot. I was immediately good on the Air Dyne and never have experienced any stress or injury from riding it. The Air Dyne also helped me use my upper body size and strength, which were actually impediments in running. In some of my aerobic routines, I do repetitions using the arm motion alone on the Air Dyne. For short repetitions (30 seconds), I have been able to "max-out," arms alone, on the Air Dyne. Using legs and arms, I can max-out for four or five minutes' duration. In the sense of a workload, maxing-out on the Air Dyne is similar to running at a five-minute pace; a running pace, of course, that I couldn't achieve.

As I added to my aerobic equipment, I had the same experience with a conventional rower, a ski machine, and power walking with weights. As soon as I started, I felt "right," and within a few sessions I was good at it. Indeed, with these activities, especially with bodybuilding, I have a very real feeling that "my body was made to do this," a feeling I never had with running. Of course, these feelings, increased abilities, and performance feedback fuel self-efficacy beliefs, outcome expectancies, and subsequent performances.

By the way, these experiences also indicate that any assessment of your aerobic capacity may depend on the type of equipment you are tested on. At this point, if I were tested on a treadmill running, I would be lucky to be in the fair range, while if I were tested for aerobic capacity on an Air Dyne, I would be in the excellent category.

When all is said and done, probably the only way you will know if you can be good at an activity or sport is to try it. Several books can help you categorize your body type and its fit with different sports, but in the end, experience and a trial period offer the best answer to the question, "What can I do and enjoy best?" By the end of two or three months, your questions will be answered, particularly if you follow the training guidelines in this book, which are reviewed and highlighted in this next section.

Motivation

After you have picked the activity (or activities) and sport you want to concentrate on, the questions you should then ask yourself should almost jump out at you after reading this book to this point. You should be systematic and analytical and ask:

- What do I want to accomplish?
- What are my specific long-term goals?

Once you can specify goals, recall that you can backtrack from an ultimate goal or simply start with a series of goals. In any case, you should end up with an ascending series of goals similar to the idea of "successive approximation" discussed in Chapter 4. After the first few goals, your goals should be hard, but realistically reachable.

Your next question should be:

- How can I within reason set up an optimal environment so that reaching my athletic and training goals is facilitated and not hindered?

For some individuals, modifying their work schedule a bit (see Chapter 2) may be very helpful. For example, a person may be able to take an extended lunch time if work time is added at the beginning or end of a day. Other people may scout out various gyms and find the one with the right clientele, equipment, and atmosphere for them. Some individuals may start developing their own home gym. The trick here is to strike a balance between the demands of the activity, your goals, and constraints on resources such as time, space, and money.

Another type of question for the novice or an individual contemplating an escalation in training is:

- What supports, incentives, and reinforcers do I need to get started, to stick with it, and to improve?

Some individuals may need, at first, a running or walking group or one training partner as a source of encouragement

and support. Other individuals may require a public commitment strategy. These individuals may like the challenge of
publicly announcing their goals or even publicly posting their
progress by displaying a cumulative chart of miles run outside
their office. Other individuals may prefer solitary training and
shun public social pressure and reinforcement. However,
these same individuals may be adept at setting up a series of
personal reinforcers for performance accomplishments.

Thinking about your likes and dislikes will lead you down a
certain motivational pathway. Once on that pathway, it is in
your hands to creatively design your own supports, incentives,
and reinforcers. For example, accomplishing an ascending series of performance goals can be attached to a series of increasingly attractive reinforcers. And, again, for some individuals, goal attainment alone will be sufficiently reinforcing.
Other questions related to prompting and monitoring performance are:

- What should my data and record keeping system
  entail?
- What aspects of performance and recovery and
  related factors should I track?
- How can these data be made simple so that it is an
  effective feedback system that I respond to?

These questions indicate that a training log should be developed to plan and record all training sessions. The log should
contain information that guides and promotes optimal performance and behavioral changes. Workouts should, for most
people, be planned in advance. The goals of each workout—
weights and repetitions, pace and distance—should follow the
periodization plan in Chapter 3. At the end of every micro-
cycle, I generally plan the next micro-cycle. And after every
week, I specifically plan and write out every workout in my log
in detail. That means, for example, that I prerecord every
weight and rep goal and then check them off as a session
proceeds. In the case of aerobics, I record after the session.

Specific comments related to accomplishment or nonaccomplishment of goals, as well as other salient points, should be noted to guide behavior change. If you notice, for example, that you always "die" on your training runs because you go out too quickly, your log should note this with a warning, such as "DIED AGAIN—MUST GO OUT SLOWLY NEXT TIME!" Obviously, log keeping is only helpful if you act on the recorded information.

I do *not* recommend that you get into elaborate computer programs. Rather, keep simple and clear records that allow you to spot short- and long-term patterns. Enhance the positive and decrease the negative feedback by understanding the data and patterns. And enjoy the satisfactions that accrue from task completion as you record your workouts in your log.

In addition, notes about self-observation processes during training are important. As we saw, all the masters athletes in this book are particularly sensitive observers of their own behavior. You can start that process by taking mental notes during training and then jotting them in your log after a session. Eventually, through trial and error and continued recording, you can develop sensitivity to the most important internal and external processes. You should be able to come up with your optimal time to train, although you might not always be able to adhere to it, and particular self-statements that alter performance, a process you can learn to optimize.

Another two questions should end this inquiry:

- How can I best make all these processes and variables—the most reasonable series of goals, enacted in certain settings, with certain supports—work together?
- And, most importantly, how can I make this entire process interesting, challenging, and *enjoyable*?

This last question again requires knowing yourself. Realistically, what do you like and not like, what are you willing and not willing to do? If you align your goals, environment, and feedback system correctly, you may find you can achieve much more than you expected with considerably more satisfaction and enjoyment than you had ever imagined!

Training

The specifics of training following the periodization model, and its fit with the psychological framework of this book, have been detailed in Chapter 3. In this section, I only want to highlight a few salient points.

I am surprised, although I shouldn't be, that many people think training must be drudgery, and that you should always kill yourself. Conversely, while I've watched some people train, I realize that they should be sitting on the couch at home. They're putting no thought or effort at all into their training.

The periodization model emphasizes a planned series of hard and easier workouts over the short- and long-term haul, with small increments in effort. For the long-term athlete used to killing himself each workout, it takes force to hold him back to 85 percent efforts. You have to try this system to convince yourself that by *not* pushing hard all the time, you will actually *surpass* all your prior performances. Likewise, enforcing the backoffs after each micro-cycle, and short, active rest periods after a macro-cycle, is absolutely necessary (see Chapter 3). The temptation is to keep pushing, and that doesn't work either.

Another key point is to always start a new exercise or routine at a *ridiculously* easy level. Many individuals push themselves so hard in the beginning that there is no room for improvement. The physical and psychological feedback becomes awful, and affect, self-efficacy beliefs, and outcome expectancies suffer.

I believe that when I start out very easily I am giving myself lots of room and time for improvement. I'm controlling the stress-recovery cycle and the feedback process.

Two examples should suffice here. Until looking at Clarence Bass's training books, I had only done dumbbell side bends a few times before. I always got very sore from this new movement and then dropped it. As I started to concentrate on bodybuilding, I knew obliques was a weak area for me, and I had to do side bends (you grasp a dumbbell in one hand and bend to that side, allowing the dumbbell to touch your foot, and return to the starting position, while also keeping your opposite hand on your head for balance and form).

This time I started with a 25-pound dumbbell and figured I had years to improve on the movement. By religiously following the periodization plan, in about four years I got to the point where I now can use a 146-pound dumbbell for the exercise during a strength cycle. That's not bad for a person with small hands, wrists, and elbows. By building up slowly, I never had any injuries with the movement.

A second example is now "in progress." For years I thought about making my squat position deeper and straighter and squatting without any knee wraps. The few times I tried to squat this way, I wouldn't concede much on the weight I used. The typical result from going to this new deep position was such incredible stiffness and pain that I could hardly walk for many days.

Then I took my own advice, swallowed some pride, and started with my new squat position by taking 100 pounds off the bar, about a 27 percent decrease in weight. The result was a perfect position and virtually no stiffness. I also quickly saw that I had a new challenge goal to achieve over the next few years. I will reach weights in my perfect squats that are 95 percent of the weights I achieved in my far-from-perfect squats.

Of course, the tables now have to be turned and the second group of individuals addressed. No one "reaches their potential" unless some of their workouts are very hard. The training variable that in the end counts the most is *intensity*. You have to really put out on your hard workouts. Follow the periodization plan, build up, keep your sessions brief, but be sure you really hit the very hard workouts you plan. Just go back and look, for example, at Barry Brown's, Barbara Filutze's, or Tracy Smith's interval sessions. That's hard training.

I can cite another example for myself. Toward the end of a micro-cycle, and especially on a leg and lower back day, when I start the routine with two sets of squats, a set of deadlifts, and a set of leg presses, I really know something. I know that in about that 12 minutes, the time it took to do those big sets, I have trained harder than most anyone around and have gotten a week's worth of effort and progress into that time. That's what it takes at the end of micro-cycle to move ahead.

POSTSCRIPT

This book will end on a more general and very positive note. We have discussed motivation, training, and athletic performance. You should now have a pretty sophisticated notion about contemporary psychology and a good idea of the different domains and factors that must be analyzed and understood to optimally enhance performance.

When we made the excursion into the arena of mental training (Chapter 4), it was quickly pointed out that the same framework we used in Chapters 2 and 3 to analyze motivation and physical training was applicable to other facets of training—the cognitive and affective aspects.

Perhaps through the text, diagrams, tables, and examples in Chapter 4, you saw that this approach and framework can be used to analyze and optimize many different kinds of behaviors. Hopefully, this book will not only encourage new perceptions of middle age, new notions of what middle-aged athletes can accomplish, and new performance levels through optimal physical and mental training programs, but also provide a framework and tools for individuals to more fully become the architects of the many potentially rich and rewarding avenues of their lives.

Appendix A
Cue-Controlled Relaxation Training

Step 1: Deep muscle relaxation training (systematically tensing and releasing 16 major muscle groups); pairing the cue word (e.g., "calm") with relaxation by silently saying the word 30–40 times, while first inhaling and as exhaling saying the cue word ("controlled breathing"); training time is about 60 minutes.

Step 2: Deep muscle relaxation training, abbreviated form, plus pairing of the cue word as above; training time is about 40 minutes.

Step 3: Everyday home practice (20–25 minutes) of more abbreviated form of relaxation training, plus pairing of the cue word as above.

Step 4: More minimal relaxation training (15 minutes), plus pairing of the cue word as above.

Step 5: Everyday home practice (10 minutes) of minimal relaxation training, plus pairing of cue word as above.

Step 6: Everyday home practice (5 minutes) of brief relaxation training, plus pairing of cue word as above.

Step 7: Use of cue word to elicit relaxation in neutral situations; repeat as needed.

Step 8: Use of cue word to elicit relaxation response based on the hierarchy of anxiety-producing-situations, working up from least to most anxiety provoking (see Chapter 4). A more difficult situation is not attempted until one that is immediately easier on the hierarchy is mastered.

References for relaxation methods:

Bernstein, D.A. and Borkovec, T.D. (1973) *Progressive Relaxation: A Manual for the Helping Professions*. Champaign, Illinois: Research Press.

Bernstein, D.A. and Given, B.A. (1984) "Progressive relaxation: Abbreviated Methods," in R.L. Woolfolk and P.N. Lehrer (Eds.): *Principles and Practice of Stress Management*. New York: Guilford Press.

Charlesworth, E.A. and Nathan, R.G. (1985) *Stress Management: A Comprehensive Guide to Wellness*. New York: Ballantine Books.

Suinn, R.M. (1986) *Seven steps to peak performance*. Toronto: Hans Huber Publishers. (Excellent step-by-step manual by well-known psychology consultant to Olympic teams. However, see parts in Chapter 4 in this book on role playing, practice, and feedback, as well as generalization and stability stages of change, areas only touched on in the manual.)

(The first two references are professional literature; the third reference is an excellent, easy to follow "how to do it" book.)

Appendix B
Bodybuilding and Aerobic Training: Performance, Exercises, Routines

The following routines are based on: Clarence Bass's *Ripped-3* and the author's "Integrative Training" article, which appeared in *Iron Man*, November, 1987.

Table One
INTEGRATIVE TRAINING SCHEDULE

	M	T	W	T	F	S	S
A.M.	High Intensity Lower Body	Walk 30 minutes	High Intensity Upper Body	Walk 30 minutes	Medium Intensity Whole Body	Walk 45 min. or Easy Aerobics	Walk 60 min.
P.M.	Medium Intensity Aerobic Exercise #1 40 minutes of interval training; more leg emphasis	Walk 30 minutes	High Intensity Aerobic Exercise #2 40 minutes of interval training; more arm emphasis	Walk 30 minutes	Easy Intensity Aerobic Exercise #3 40 minutes of interval training		

278

TABLE TWO
INTEGRATIVE TRAINING SCHEDULE #2

Week One

	M	T	W	T	F	S	S
A.M.	High Intensity Lower Body	Walk 30 min.	High Intensity Upper Body	Walk 30 min.	Medium Intensity Lower Body	Walk 45 min. or Easy Aerobics	Walk 60 min.
P.M.	Medium Intensity Aerobic Exercise #1 40 min. of interval training; more leg emphasis		High Intensity Aerobic Exercise #2 40 min. of interval training; more arm emphasis		Easy Intensity Aerobic Exercise #3 40 min. of interval training		

Week Two

	M	T	W	T	F	S	S
A.M.	High Intensity Upper Body	Walk 30 min.	High Intensity Lower Body	Walk 30 min.	Medium Intensity Upper Body	Walk 45 min. or Easy Aerobics	Walk 60 min.
P.M.	Medium Intensity Aerobic exercise #1 w/ more arm emphasis		High Intensity Aerobic Exercise #2 w/ more leg emphasis		Easy Intensity Aerobic Exer. #3		

TABLE THREE
INTEGRATIVE SCHEDULE #3

	M	T	W	Th	F	S	S
A.M.	High Intensity Chest, Back, Upper Abs	High Intensity Legs, Lower Back, Obliques	High Intensity Shoulders, Arms, Lower Abs	Walk 45 Minutes	Medium Intensity Whole Body	Walk 45 Minutes	Walk 60 Minutes
P.M.	High Intensity Air Dyne, Arm Emphasis, 40 minutes	Medium Intensity, Power Walking or cycling, 40 minutes	Medium Intensity, Rowing 40 minutes		Easy Intensity Ski Machine 40 minutes		

TABLE FOUR
A PERIODIZATION APPROACH
(4-week periods)

Period	Bodybuilding	Aerobics
"Endurance"	Main exercises in sets of 15–25 reps; other exercises, 20 reps; slower, continuous reps	Moderate repetitions of 2–4 minutes; shorter intervals between repetitions*
"Strength & Endurance"	Main exercises in sets of 10–15 reps; other exercises, 12 reps; moderate speed reps with pause	Moderate to hard repetitions of 1–4 minutes; moderate intervals between repetitions*
"Strength"	Main exercises in sets of 6–10 reps; other exercises, 8 reps; fast but controlled reps with pause	Hard repetitions of ¼ to 2 minutes; long intervals between repetitions*

*During intervals, continue the exercise at an easy or moderate pace.

Table Five
EXAMPLE OF EXERCISES, SETS, AND REPETITIONS FOR TWO BODY PARTS DURING A STRENGTH/ENDURANCE PHASE

Body Part	Exercise	Sets	Reps	Warm-up Sets	Reps
upper back	T-BAR Rows	2	10,15	3	5–2
	Close Grip Chins	2	10,15	1	3
	Cable Rows	1	12	1	3
	Dumbbell Pullover	1	12	1	3
	Wide Grip Pulldowns	1	12	1	3
		7		7	
thighs	Squats	2	10,15	4	10–3
	Leg Extension	2	10,15	2	5–3
	Leg Press	1	10–12	2	5–3
	Hack Squat	1	10–12	1	3
		6		9	

BIBLIOGRAPHY

Antonovski, A. (1987). *Unraveling the Mystery of Health*. San Francisco: Jossey Bass.

Bandura, A. (1986). *Social Foundations of Thought and Action: A Social Cognitive Theory*. Englewood Cliffs: Prentice Hall.

Bass, C. (1986). *Ripped-3: The Recipes, the Routines, and the Reasons*. Albuquerque: Ripped Enterprises.

Bass, C. (1984). *The Lean Advantage*. Albuquerque: Ripped Enterprises.

Bass, C. (1982). *Ripped-2*. Albuquerque: Ripped Enterprises.

Bass, C. (1980). *Ripped*. Albuquerque: Ripped Enterprises.

Brooks, G. A. and Fahey, T. D. (1984). *Exercise Physiology: Human Bioenergetics and its Applications*. New York: Wiley.

Brownell, K. D., Marlatt, A., Lichtenstein, E., and Wilson, G. T. (1986). Understanding and Preventing Relapse. *American Psychologist, 41*, 765–782.

Cooper, K. H. (1982). *The Aerobics Program for Total Well-Being*. New York: M. Evans and Company, Inc.

Hatfield, B. D. and Walford, G. A. (1987). "Understanding Anxiety: Implications for Sports Performance." *National Strength and Conditioning Association Journal, 9(2)*, 58–65.

Hatfield, F. C. (1984). *Bodybuilding: A Scientific Approach*. Chicago: Contemporary

Hickson, R. C., Foster, C., Pollock, M. L., Galassi, T. M., and Rich, S. (1985). Reduced Training Intensities and Loss of Aerobic Power, Endurance, and Cardiac Growth. *Journal of Applied Physiology, 58*, 492–499.

Jerome, J. (1984). *Staying with It: On Becoming an Athlete.* New York: Viking Penguin, Inc.

Kahn, Jr., L. (1986). *Over the Hill: But Not Out to Lunch.* Bolinas, CA: Shelter Publications, Inc.

Paffenbarger, R. S., Hyde, R. T., Wing, A. L., and Hseih, C. (1986). Physical Activity, All-Cause Mortality, and Longevity of College Alumni. *New England Journal of Medicine, 314*, 605–613.

Pearl, B. (1982). *Keys to the Inner Universe.* Phoenix, OR: Bill Pearl Enterprises.

Pearl, B. and Moran, G. T. (1986). *Getting Stronger.* Bolinas, CA: Shelter Publications, Inc. .

Pollock, M. L., Foster, C., Knapp, D., Rod, J. L., and Schmidt, D. H. (1987). "Effect of Age, Training, and Competition on Aerobic Capacity and Body Composition of Masters Athletes. *Journal of Applied Physiology. 63*, 725–31.

Pollock, M. L., Wilmore, J. H., and Fox III, S. M. (1984). *Exercise in Health and Disease: Evaluation and Prescription for Prevention and Rehabilitation.* Philadelphia: W. B. Saunders Company.

Stone, M. H. and O'Bryant, H. S. (1984). *Weight Training: A Scientific Approach* (preliminary edition). Minneapolis: Burgers Publishing Company.

Suinn, R. M. (1987). *Seven Steps to Peak Performance.* New York: Hans Huber Publishers.

Todd, J. and Todd, T. (1985). *Lift your Way to Youthful Fitness.* Boston: Little, Brown, & Company.

Walford, R. L. (1986). *Maximum Life Span.* New York: W. W. Norton & Co.

Index

285